Cardiovascular Disease

Editor

MARK B. STEPHENS

PRIMARY CARE:
CLINICS IN OFFICE PRACTICE

www.primarycare.theclinics.com

Consulting Editor
JOEL J. HEIDELBAUGH

March 2018 • Volume 45 • Number 1

ELSEVIER

1600 John F. Kennedy Boulevard • Suite 1800 • Philadelphia, Pennsylvania, 19103-2899

http://www.theclinics.com

PRIMARY CARE: CLINICS IN OFFICE PRACTICE Volume 45, Number 1
March 2018 ISSN 0095-4543, ISBN-13: 978-0-323-58166-0

Editor: Jessica McCool
Developmental Editor: Laura Fisher

Primary Care: Clinics in Office Practice (ISSN: 0095-4543) is published quarterly by Elsevier Inc., 360 Park Avenue South, New York, NY 10010-1710. Months of issue are March, June, September, and December. Periodicals postage paid at New York, NY and additional mailing offices. Subscription prices are $237.00 per year (US individuals), $474.00 (US institutions), $100.00 (US students), $289.00 (Canadian individuals), $536.00 (Canadian institutions), $175.00 (Canadian students), $355.00 (international individuals), $536.00 (international institutions), and $175.00 (international students). Foreign air speed delivery is included in all *Clinics* subscription prices. All prices are subject to change without notice. POSTMASTER: Send address changes to *Primary Care: Clinics in Office Practice*, Elsevier Periodicals Customer Service, 11830 Westline Industrial Drive, St. Louis, MO 63146. Customer Service Health Sciences Division, Subscription Customer Service, 3251 Riverport Lane, Maryland Heights, MO 63043. **Customer Service: 1-800-654-2452 (U.S. and Canada); 314-447-8871 (outside U.S. and Canada). Fax: 314-447-8029. E-mail: journalscustomerservice-usa@elsevier.com (for print support); journalsonlinesupport-usa@elsevier.com (for online support).**

Reprints. For copies of 100 or more, of articles in this publication, please contact the Commercial Reprints Department, Elsevier Inc., 360 Park Avenue South, New York, NY 10010-1710. Tel. 212-633-3874; Fax: 212-633-3820; E-mail: reprints@elsevier.com.

Primary Care: Clinics in Office Practice is covered in *MEDLINE/PubMed (Index Medicus)* and *EMBASE/Excerpta Medica, Current Contents/Clinical Medicine,* and *ISI/BIOMED*.

Contributors

CONSULTING EDITOR

JOEL J. HEIDELBAUGH, MD, FAAFP, FACG
Clinical Professor, Departments of Family Medicine and Urology; University of Michigan Medical School, Ann Arbor, Michigan

EDITOR

MARK B. STEPHENS, MD
Professor of Family and Community Medicine, Penn State University College of Medicine, State College, Pennsylvania

AUTHORS

JARED L. ANTEVIL, MD, FACS
Associate Professor, Department of Surgery, Division of Cardiothoracic Surgery, Uniformed Services University of the Health Sciences, Walter Reed National Military Medical Center, Bethesda, Maryland

MICHAEL BERGE, MD
Diagnostic Radiology Resident, National Capital Consortium, Walter Reed National Military Medical Center, Bethesda, Maryland

STEPHEN D. CAGLE Jr, MD
Assistant Professor Family Medicine, O'Fallon, Highland, Illinois

KEITH A. CLAUSSEN, DO
Eastern Virginia Medical School, Norfolk, Virginia

NOAH COOPERSTEIN, MD
O'Fallon, Belleville, Illinois

RON DOMMERMUTH, MD
Faculty, Northwest Washington Family Medicine Residency, Bremerton, Washington

KRISTINE EWING, MD
Staff Physician, Department of Family Medicine, Naval Hospital Bremerton, Bremerton, Washington

ANDREW J. FOY, MD
Assistant Professor of Medicine and Public Health Sciences, Cardiology Division, Penn State College of Medicine, Hershey, Pennsylvania

RICHARD U. GARCIA, MD
Division of Cardiac Critical Care Medicine, Departments of Pediatrics and Critical Care Medicine, The University of Pennsylvania, The Children's Hospital of Philadelphia, Philadelphia, Pennsylvania

JEFFERY T. GRAY, MD
Internal Medicine Residency, Department of Medicine, Walter Reed National Military Medical Center, Bethesda, Maryland

BRIAN A. HEMANN, MD, FACC
Associate Professor, Department of Medicine, Uniformed Services University of the Health Sciences, Chief of Medicine, Walter Reed National Military Medical Center, Bethesda, Maryland

VINCENT B. HO, MD, MBA
Chief, Department of Radiology, Walter Reed National Military Medical Center, Chair and Professor, Department of Radiology and Radiological Sciences, Uniformed Services University of the Health Sciences, Bethesda, Maryland

MAUREEN N. HOOD, PhD
Assistant Professor, Department of Radiology and Radiological Sciences, Uniformed Services University of the Health Sciences, Nurse Scientist, Walter Reed National Military Medical Center, Bethesda, Maryland

SCOTT P. HOPKINS, MD, FACC
Assistant Professor, Department of Medicine, Division of Cardiology, Uniformed Services University of the Health Sciences, Walter Reed National Military Medical Center, Bethesda, Maryland

DANIEL P. KUCKEL, MD, MS, MBA, LCDR, MC, USN
Chief Resident of Family Medicine, Naval Hospital Jacksonville, Jacksonville, Florida

KARL A. KUERSTEINER, MD
Naval Hospital Jacksonville, Jacksonville, Florida

KYLE P. LAMMLEIN, MD
Resident Physician, Family Medicine, National Capital Consortium Family Medicine Residency, Fort Belvoir Community Hospital, Fort Belvoir, Virginia

ROBERT P. LENNON, MD, JD, FAAFP
Naval Hospital Jacksonville, Jacksonville, Florida

ELIZABETH ANNE LEONARD, MD
Associate Program Director, United States Navy, Camp Lejeune Family Medicine Residency, Camp Lejeune, North Carolina; Assistant Professor of Family Medicine, Uniformed Services University of the Health Sciences, Bethesda, Maryland

JOHN P. LICHTENBERGER III, MD
Associate Professor, Department of Radiology and Radiological Sciences, Uniformed Services University of the Health Sciences, Bethesda, Maryland

JOHN M. MANDROLA, MD
Cardiologist, Louisville Cardiology Group at Baptist Health, Louisville, Kentucky

ROBERT JAMES MARSHALL, MD
CardioCare, LLC, Assistant Professor of Medicine, The George Washington University Hospital, Washington, DC

ZORANA MRSIC, MD
Instructor, Department of Medicine, Division of Cardiology, Uniformed Services University of the Health Sciences, Walter Reed National Military Medical Center, Bethesda, Maryland

PHILIP S. MULLENIX, MD, FACS, FCCP
Associate Professor, Department of Surgery, Division of Cardiothoracic Surgery, Uniformed Services University of the Health Sciences, Walter Reed National Military Medical Center, Bethesda, Maryland

BRIAN E. NEUBAUER, MD, FACP
Assistant Professor, Department of Medicine, Uniformed Services University of the Health Sciences, Chief, General Internal Medicine Service, Department of Medicine, Walter Reed National Military Medical Center, Bethesda, Maryland

FRANCIS G. O'CONNOR, MD, MPH
Professor and Chair, Department of Military and Emergency Medicine, Uniformed Services University of the Health Sciences, Bethesda, Maryland

STACIE B. PEDDY, MD
Division of Cardiac Critical Care Medicine, Departments of Pediatrics and Critical Care Medicine, The University of Pennsylvania, The Children's Hospital of Philadelphia, Philadelphia, Pennsylvania

PAUL GABRIEL PETERSON, MD
Chief of Cardiothoracic Imaging, Department of Radiology, Walter Reed National Military Medical Center, Assistant Professor, Department of Radiology and Radiological Sciences, Uniformed Services University of the Health Sciences, Bethesda, Maryland

BRIAN V. REAMY, MD
Senior Associate Dean for Academic and Faculty Affairs, Professor of Family Medicine and Medicine, F. Edward Hébert School of Medicine, Uniformed Services University, Bethesda, Maryland

JONATHAN M. STODDARD, MD
Resident Physician, Family Medicine, National Capital Consortium Family Medicine Residency, Fort Belvoir Community Hospital, Fort Belvoir, Virginia

PAMELA M. WILLIAMS, MD, Colonel, USAF, MC
Director of Medical Education, Mike O'Callaghan Federal Medical Center, Nellis AFB, Nevada; Associate Professor of Family Medicine, F. Edward Hébert School of Medicine, Uniformed Services University, Bethesda, Maryland

Contents

> Cardiovascular diseases are prevalent worldwide and have significant impact on morbidity, mortality, and overall health care costs. Common risk factors include obesity, hypertension, hyperlipidemia, diabetes mellitus, chronic kidney disease, and smoking. Both modifiable and nonmodifiable risks should be accounted for when evaluating and managing patients with cardiovascular diseases. The complex nature of cardiovascular disease is not fully understood. Therefore, primary care physicians must balance what is known, what is suspected, and each patient's individual preferences to create an optimal treatment plan.

> The United States spends more on health care than any other industrialized nation. In 2016, health care expenditure reached an estimated $3.35 trillion or $10,345 per individual. Cardiovascular disease represents the leading cause of death and disability as well as the most significant source of health care spending. This article reviews the current economic burden of heart disease in the United States, presents future projections, and explores factors driving cost growth in cardiovascular care.

> Cardiovascular disease remains the leading cause of death in the United States and worldwide. Prevention of cardiovascular disease is an achievable goal. A rigorous 2010 analysis by the World Health Organization suggests that reducing risk factors in young adults and maintaining an optimum risk profile through age 50 years could prevent 90% of atherosclerotic cardiovascular disease events. Misinformation and poor implementation of proven preventive strategies, misplaced fears of medications, or incorrect understanding of ideal dietary and lifestyle choices all contribute to poor risk profiles. Every patient deserves an individualized prescription for cardiovascular disease prevention incorporating strategies to control modifiable cardiovascular risk factors.

Metabolic syndrome (MetS) is a cluster of cardiometabolic risk factors. MetS is associated with an approximately 4-fold increase in the likelihood of developing type 2 diabetes mellitus (T2DM) and a 2-fold increase in the incidence of cardiovascular disease complications. MetS is a progressive, proinflammatory, prothrombotic condition that manifests itself along a broad spectrum of disease. It is associated with hypertension, obstructive sleep apnea, fatty liver disease, gout, and polycystic ovarian syndrome. Intervening in and reversing the pathologic process become more difficult as the disease progresses, highlighting the needs for increased individual and community surveillance and primary prevention.

Cardiovascular disease in women as a distinct disease entity is underappreciated relative to other female-specific diseases. A perception that cardiovascular disease affects men more commonly and a lack of understanding about the underlying pathophysiology of cardiovascular disease in women contribute to this phenomenon. Hormonal changes, pregnancy-related conditions, and cancer therapies have an impact on endothelial function, vascular anatomy, and myocardial contractility. Women with heart disease often present later, receive care not consistent with accepted guidelines, and have less access to diagnostic and therapeutic resources. Understanding the differences and challenges of treating cardiovascular disease in women is essential to improving population health.

The pediatric cardiology field has developed rapidly over the past few decades. More children than ever born with congenital heart disease (CHD) are growing into adulthood. Primary care providers play a key role in diagnosis, management, and referral of children with CHD because many common cardiac complaints (eg, feeding intolerance, cyanosis, chest pain, palpitations, and syncope) are first addressed in the primary care setting. The spectrum of heart disease in children ranges from common complaints to complex single-ventricle physiology, acute myocarditis, and heart transplantation. This article reviews the pathophysiology and management of the most frequent cardiac conditions encountered in primary care.

 Video content accompanies this article at http://www.primarycare. theclinics.com.

Cardiovascular imaging with calcium scoring computed tomography (CT), coronary CT angiography (CCTA), and cardiac MRI (CMR) have advanced rapidly over recent years. These imaging modalities have increased in availability, accessibility, and clinical practicality owing to technologic advances allowing for significant radiation dose reduction for high-quality CCTA and for rapid and reliable imaging techniques in CMR. Hardware and software developments are continually increasing efficiency and accuracy of postprocessing. In the context of these rapidly developing imaging modalities, it is critical for ordering physicians and providers to be aware of the fundamentals of each modality, imaging challenges, and appropriate use criteria.

PRIMARY CARE:
CLINICS IN OFFICE PRACTICE

ISSUE OF RELATED INTEREST

Physician Assistant Clinics, October 2017 (Vol. 2, No. 4)
Cardiology
Daniel T. Thibodeau, *Editor*
Available at: http://www.physicianassistant.theclinics.com/

THE CLINICS ARE AVAILABLE ONLINE!
Access your subscription at:
www.theclinics.com

Foreword

The Price of the Heart

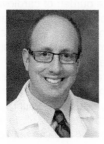

Joel J. Heidelbaugh, MD, FAAFP, FACG
Consulting Editor

In a recent wellness examination on a late-middle-aged man whom I've known for almost 2 decades, my patient asked, *"Can you just order all of the blood tests for cancer screening so that I can go?"* His goal was to get in and out of my office as quickly as possible so that he could go to the gym before meeting his wife later that evening for her birthday dinner. As a reasonably healthy nonsmoking and moderate alcohol-consuming patient with only well-controlled hypertension and hyperlipidemia as his medical issues, I courageously explained that his wellness exam encompassed much more than just cancer screening. He wasn't interested in immunizations, discussions about nutrition or sleep, and because cholesterol values were normal 3 years ago (on a statin) and his current blood pressure was normal (on a thiazide diuretic, a calcium channel blocker, and an angiotensin converting enzyme inhibitor), his hopes were to get "in and out." Perhaps ironically, I realized in reviewing his chart that while I had ordered relevant laboratory tests each of the last few years, they were not obtained.

On a thorough review of systems, I learned that while his hypertension and hyperlipidemia were well controlled, his diet generally consisted of sugars and carbohydrates with few fruits and vegetables, modest protein, and snacks high in saturated fats. Moreover, while he admitted to exercising several times per week, he commented that his elliptical trainer workouts have gotten "shorter and shorter" because he "sweats heavier and heavier" and thought his symptoms were due to poor sleep from work stress. He also admitted to recent presyncopal symptoms after climbing stairs. Recognizing that his parents (both of whom are my patients) have coronary artery disease, I recommended a cardiac stress test that week and that he hold off on vigorous exercise. My patient seemed rather surprised and remarked, "I get a stress test every time I work out, doc. I don't need to do that. Plus, we don't need to do an expensive test that will be normal." After a more detailed conversation, my patient did agree to a stress test, which proved to be abnormal and resulted in a cardiac catheterization and stent placement in his left anterior descending artery, which was 70%

occluded. In follow-up, my patient was thankful for my persistence in guiding him to undergo a cardiac stress test. In hindsight, he commented that *"the price of his heart was worth more than anything money could buy his family."*

This issue of *Primary Care: Clinics in Office Practice* encompasses the most important tenets of cardiovascular disease management that we encounter in daily practice. The issue commences with an in-depth examination of the burden of cardiovascular diseases from both epidemiologic and economic perspectives. As heart disease remains the number one killer of men and women in the United States, it remains our ultimate goal to minimize morbidity and mortality. Prevention, diagnosis, and evidence-based management of coronary artery disease, congestive heart failure, and valvular heart disease remain paramount, while challenging when guidelines change often. The preparticipation sports physical examination remains on the forefront of all of our minds when we evaluate commonly asymptomatic young athletes who may be predisposed to an undetected condition that may result in sudden cardiac death. Cardiometabolic syndrome remains an enigmatic entity to both characterize and treat, while heart disease in women and children often goes underappreciated and underevaluated. Last, cardiac imaging is a rapidly advancing area of medicine that primary care clinicians will need to utilize and interpret.

I would like to thank Dr Mark B. Stephens, one of our seasoned guest editors, for compiling another outstanding collection of relevant review articles for this issue of *Primary Care: Clinics in Office Practice* dedicated to cardiovascular diseases. These disorders remain central to our everyday practices and the patients we care for. I hope that you will find this issue as enlightening and instructive as I have.

Joel J. Heidelbaugh, MD, FAAFP, FACG
Departments of Family Medicine and Urology
University of Michigan Medical School
Ann Arbor, MI 48103, USA

Ypsilanti Health Center
200 Arnet, Suite 200
Ypsilanti, MI 48198, USA

E-mail address:
jheidel@umich.edu

Preface

Be Still My Beating Heart: Cardiovascular Disease in the United States

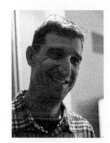

Mark B. Stephens, MD
Editor

Cardiovascular disease remains the leading cause of death for Americans. When examining what factors contribute to the premature stilling of too many heartbeats, it is clear that lifestyle factors (specifically physical activity patterns and dietary habits) play a central role. Despite explosive advances in pharmacology and medical imaging, the most important prescription available in modern medicine to promote health and well-being remains adequate physical activity. When coupled with healthy eating habits, the dynamic duo of diet and activity are powerful crusaders of prevention.

This issue of *Primary Care: Clinics in Office Practice* is dedicated to an in-depth look at cardiovascular disease through the lens of primary care. Health systems science is of growing interest in medical education and health care delivery. With this in mind, the initial articles focus on epidemiology, economics, and prevention of cardiovascular disease from the perspective of individual patients to population health. Subsequent articles focus on more traditional topics within cardiovascular medicine. Coronary artery disease, congestive heart failure, and valvular heart disease deal with supply, demand, and pump function. Primary care physicians and advanced practitioners are at the front line of recognition and treatment of each of these conditions.

Sudden cardiac death (SCD) has intermittently grabbed headlines in high-profile athletes. Screening athletes for SCD is an important primary care role. Knowing who can safely compete and who needs referral is an objective of this issue that can be put to immediate practice. We return to systems thinking with an approach to metabolic syndrome. Representing a cluster of conditions manifested by increases in blood pressure, blood sugar, serum lipids, weight and waist circumference, a systems approach to metabolic syndrome requires different approaches in the setting of the patient-centered medical home.

Prim Care Clin Office Pract 45 (2018) xv–xvi
https://doi.org/10.1016/j.pop.2017.12.002
0095-4543/18/© 2017 Published by Elsevier Inc.

The issue continues with articles reviewing heart disease in women and children. Cardiovascular disease can have atypical presentations in each of these populations. These articles are dedicated to issues unique to women and children in terms of diagnosis and management. The issue concludes with a review of cardiac imaging. With the increasing array of imaging modalities, it is important that primary care physicians know the indications, risks, and benefits of those currently available.

After reviewing the available science in the ever-changing world of cardiovascular medicine, a key take-away message from this issue remains the central importance of sound dietary and physical activity habits in the prevention and treatment of cardiovascular disease. Keep moving, my beating heart; there is still much work to be done.

Mark B. Stephens, MD
Penn State University College of Medicine
1850 East Park Avenue
Suite 207
State College, PA 16803, USA

E-mail address:
mstephens3@pennstatehealth.psu.edu

State of the Heart

An Overview of the Disease Burden of Cardiovascular Disease from an Epidemiologic Perspective

Robert P. Lennon, MD, JD[a],*, Keith A. Claussen, DO[b], Karl A. Kuersteiner, MD[c]

KEYWORDS

- Cardiovascular disease • Hypertension • Obesity • Hyperlipidemia
- Diabetes mellitus • Chronic kidney disease

KEY POINTS

- Cardiovascular diseases are present in all human populations and significantly impact health.
- Cardiovascular diseases have multiple synergistic causes requiring a comprehensive approach to their diagnosis and treatment.
- Early intervention is a cornerstone of management.

INTRODUCTION

Although preventable, cardiovascular disease (CVD) remains the leading cause of death worldwide. This article discusses the state of the heart from an epidemiologic perspective, reviewing the definition of CVD, associated risk factors, global health impact, and correlation to clinical practice. See **Box 1** for a definition of CVDs.

Disclosure: The authors have no commercial or financial conflicts of interest. The authors were not funded for this project.

Disclaimer: The views expressed in this article are those of the authors and do not necessarily reflect the official policy or position of the Department of the Navy, Department of Defense, or the United States Government.

Copyright Statement: The authors are military service members. This work was prepared as part of our official duties. Title 17 U.S C. 105 provides that "Copyright protection under this title is not available for any work of the United States Government." Title 17 U.S C. 101 defines United States Government work as a work prepared by a military service member or employee of the United States Government as part of that person's official duties.

[a] Naval Hospital Jacksonville, Jacksonville, FL 32214, USA; [b] Eastern Virginia Medical School, Norfolk, VA 23507, USA; [c] Naval Hospital Jacksonville, Jacksonville, FL 32214, USA
* Corresponding author.
E-mail address: Robert.p.lennon.mil@mail.mil

> **Box 1**
> **Definition of cardiovascular disease**
>
> CVD is a group of disorders of the heart and blood vessels, including coronary heart disease, cerebrovascular disease, peripheral artery disease, rheumatic heart disease, congenital heart disease, deep vein thrombosis, and pulmonary embolism.
>
> *Data from* World Health Organization. Cardiovascular disease. 2017. Available at: http://www.who.int/cardiovascular_diseases/about_cvd/en/. Accessed December 15, 2017.

RISK FACTORS

Risk factors for CVD are numerous and additive; acute forms such as heart attacks and strokes often occur in the presence of multiple risk factors. Risk factors are often categorized broadly as modifiable and nonmodifiable. However, as more risk factors are uncovered, some may more accurately be described as maybe modifiable.

Nonmodifiable Risk Factors

Eighty percent of all CVD mortality occurs in patients older than the age of 65 years (**Box 2**). Men older than 45 and women older than the age of 55 years are generally considered to be at higher risk of death from CVD. The gender benefit of lower CVD rates decreases after menopause.[1] CVD is higher in non-Hispanic whites, non-Hispanic blacks, and American Indians.[2] In the United States, the CVD death rate for black men is 53% higher and the death rate for black women is 8% higher than the overall CVD death rate.[3] Family history refers to CVD in a first-degree male relative before age 55 years or a first-degree female relative before age 65 years.[4] The "My Family Health Portrait" Web site (https://familyhistory.hhs.gov/FHH/html/index.html) is a useful tool for exploring family history.

Maybe Modifiable Risk Factors

There are several socioeconomic factors that are potentially modifiable. Specifically, ischemic heart disease and stroke are inversely related to education, income, and poverty status.[5] The mortality benefit from reduced CVD from improved socioeconomic conditions is a driving factor behind modern public health programs and presents a strong argument for investing in health infrastructure.

> **Box 2**
> **Nonmodifiable and maybe modifiable risk factors for cardiovascular disease**
>
> *Nonmodifiable*
>
> Age
>
> Male Gender
>
> Ethnicity
>
> Family history
>
> *Maybe modifiable*
>
> Education level
>
> Income
>
> Poverty status

Modifiable Risk Factors

The importance of identifying and addressing modifiable risk factors (**Box 3**) early was clearly demonstrated in the Framingham Heart Study, which showed that the absence of established risk factors at 50 years of age is associated with low lifetime CVD risks and improved long-term survival.[6]

There is a significant and linear increase in the relative risk of ischemic heart disease for individuals who smoke between 1 and 5 cigarettes to those who smoke from 5 to 30 cigarettes per day.[7] Cumulative tobacco use also increases CVD risk per decade when examined according to the number of cigarettes per day, age, and number of years smoked.[8] In addition, second-hand smoke increases CVD risk as much as 30%.[9]

Obesity and overweight are independent risk factors for CVD. Relative risk of CVD for obese patients increases 46% for men and 64% for women. Being overweight increases the relative risk of CVD 21% for men and 20% for women.[10,11] When used in isolation, however, body mass index (BMI) is not a reliable risk predictor. The importance of abdominal obesity is increasingly recognized. A subgroup of obese patients, the metabolically healthy obese, have a CVD risk that is higher than normal-weight patients but lower than expected based on BMI alone.[12] This highlights the importance of physical activity in the prevention of CVD.

Sedentary lifestyle is an independent risk factor for CVD in both men and women. Physical activity improves CVD mortality in both healthy subjects and those with metabolic risk factors.[13] Moderate intensity physical activity for 150 minutes per week lowers CVD risk by 14%. Increasing to 300 minutes per week of moderate physical activity lowers CVD risk by 20%.[14]

Poor dietary habits also contribute directly to CVD risk. The importance of ingesting a healthful, food-based diet is increasingly recognized. Diets that focus on individual nutrient targets (ie, low-fat or low-saturated fat diets) consistently fail to demonstrate a sustained positive effect on CVD risk. The optimal diet for CVD health is one with minimal intake of refined carbohydrates, processed meats, and foods high in sodium and trans fat. Patients should aim for a moderate intake of unprocessed red meats, poultry, eggs, and milk. Fruits, nuts, fish, vegetables (excluding russet or white potatoes), vegetable oils, minimally processed whole grains, legumes, and yogurt are recommended in higher quantities.[15]

Box 3
Modifiable risk factors for cardiovascular disease

Modifiable

Tobacco use

Second-hand smoke

Obesity or overweight

Sedentary lifestyle

Poor diet

Excessive alcohol

Hypertension

DM or pre-DM

Hyperlipidemia

Stress

Light to moderate alcohol consumption during middle age is associated with lower CVD risk in both men and women. The causality of this association and significant concern regarding other risks of alcohol consumption make this recommendation controversial. Consumption of alcohol in excess of 40g per day yields higher rates of CVD. The American Heart Association (AHA) does not recommend alcohol consumption for heart health, and advises individuals to drink only in moderation: 1 to 2 drinks per day for men and 1 drink per day for women (a drink is 12 ounces of beer, 4 ounces of wine, 1.5 ounces of 80-proof spirits, or 1 ounce of 100-proof spirits).[16,17]

For all ages and genders, CVD risk increases with blood pressure even within normal ranges.[18] The Eighth Joint National Committee recommends that adults 18 to 60 years of age maintain a blood pressure lower than 140/90, adults 60 years and older maintain a blood pressure lower than 150/90, and adults of all ages with diabetes mellitus (DM) or chronic kidney disease (CKD) maintain a blood pressure lower than 140/90.[19]

DM is a well-established risk factor for CVD. Optimal glycemic control (in addition to control of comorbid risks) improves CVD risk in diabetics. This benefit is greatest with early intervention.[20]

Hyperlipidemia is also associated with an increased risk of CVD. Currently, treatment with medication (statin therapy) is based on calculated risk. There are several online risk calculators, including http://www.cvriskcalculator.com, which estimate risk based on the 2013 American College of Cardiology (ACC) and AHA guideline on the assessment of cardiovascular risk.[21] Treatment is recommended for primary prevention in patients whose 10-year CVD risk is greater than or equal to 7.5%. Patients with a lower risk may also be candidates for statin therapy (5% to <7.5% 10-year CVD risk, low-density lipoprotein cholesterol [LDL-C] levels greater than or equal to 160 mg/dL, strong family history of premature CVD, elevated lifetime CVD risk, abnormal coronary artery calcification score or ankle-brachial index, or high-sensitivity C-reactive protein $\geq$2 mg/L). Diabetics, individuals with other clinical manifestations of CVD, and patients with LDL-C greater than or equal to 190 mg/dL are also candidates for statin therapy.[22]

Emotional stress has emerged as a risk factor for CVD. Although the association is not yet well understood, short-term emotional stress is known to trigger acute CVD events, and long-term stress is associated with increased recurrent CVD events.[23] Stress has been shown to have CVD risk gradients comparable to elevated cholesterol and stress intervention programs have shown positive results in terms of risk and disease reduction.[24]

PREVALENCE OR INCIDENCE

CVDs, cancers, and mental health and substance use disorders are the predominant sources of noncommunicable disease (NCD) worldwide.[25] NCD now accounts for 2 out of 3 deaths worldwide (Fig. 1).[26] CVD is the leading cause of mortality, singularly responsible for 30% of all global deaths (Fig. 2).[27,28] Coronary heart disease alone causes 19% of deaths among men and 20% among women. This is triple the number of male deaths attributable to lung cancer and nearly10 times the number of female deaths from breast cancer. Coronary heart disease and cerebrovascular disease together constitute approximately 80% of total CVD mortality.[25,29] The total global impact of CVD results in twice as many deaths as cancer, and more than all communicable diseases, maternal and neonatal disorders, and nutritional disorders combined.[27]

As CVD established itself as the leading cause of death in the developed world during the twentieth century, high-income countries achieved substantial reductions in

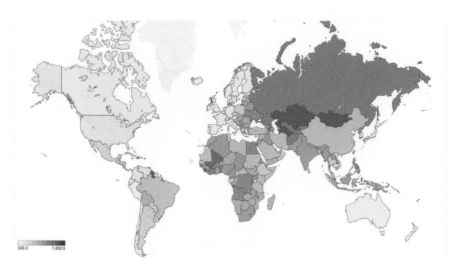

Fig. 1. 2012: NCD age-standardized mortality rate (per 100,000). (*Data from* World Health Organization; available at: http://www.who.int/gho/en/.)

CVD mortality through coordinated preventive efforts.[28,30,31] As a result, first-time hospitalization for myocardial infarction has decreased by 50% and mortality rates from cerebrovascular disease have decreased 37% to 45% in the Western world since the 1980s (**Figs. 3** and **4**).[32,33] In the last decade, the incidence of myocardial infarction and stroke in developed countries has decreased by almost one-third.[34] Primary preventive efforts targeting reductions in untreated blood pressure, smoking, and sedentary lifestyle, combined with aggressive medical and procedural treatment, has led to this decline.[32,35–37] Due to advances in CVD prevention and treatment, most regions of the globe have seen declines in CVD age-specific death rates (**Fig. 5**). Improvements in cardiovascular health have resulted in nearly 2 million fewer deaths from coronary

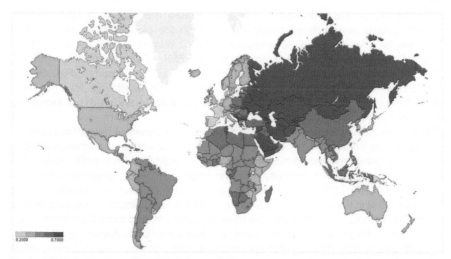

Fig. 2. 2012: Proportion of NCD death rate due to CVD. (*Data from* World Health Organization; available at: http://www.who.int/gho/en/.)

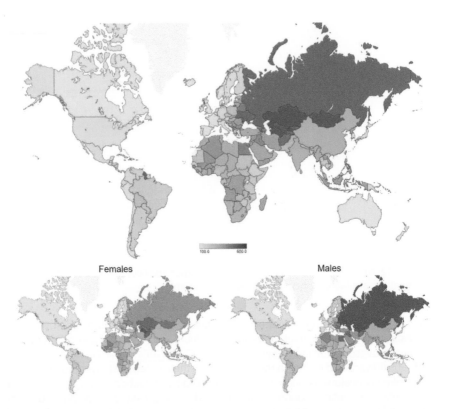

Fig. 3. 2012: CVD age-standardized mortality rate (per 100,000). (*Data from* World Health Organization; available at: http://www.who.int/gho/en/.)

heart disease alone worldwide since 1990 based on predicted age-specific death rate.[37]

Despite impressive improvements in CVD-related mortality, population growth and aging have overwhelmed these advances on the global scale. These trends have resulted in an absolute increase in CVD-related death by 40% since 1990.[28,37] Regional trends have emerged with 75% of the premature mortality from CVD now borne by low-income and middle-income countries (**Fig. 6**).[38] In sub-Saharan Africa, for example, the CVD age-specific death rate was generally stable from 1990 to 2013, but the absolute number of CVD deaths increased 81% over the same period.[28]

Other noteworthy trends in CVD-related mortality are evident in developing nations. In India, where undernutrition, infectious diseases, and maternal and neonatal diseases were previously predominant drivers of mortality and morbidity, CVDs are now the leading cause of mortality.[29,39] The impact of CVD is predominantly seen earlier in life (52% of CVD-related deaths occur before 70 years of age) and there is a linear increase in the risk of CVD associated with the rising prevalence of established risk factors. In India, 35% of adults use tobacco products, 1 of every 2 adults is physically inactive, diets have less than 1 serving of fruit a week, and hypertension rates in adults approach 30%.[29] Some of these cardiovascular risks are predicted to be offset by improved sanitation, decreased household air pollution, accessibility of clean water,[40] and access to cost-effective treatments such as blood-pressure and

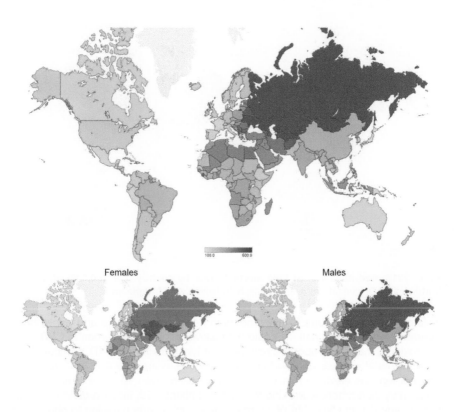

Fig. 4. 2000: CVD age-standardized mortality rate (per 100,000). (*Data from* World Health Organization; available at: http://www.who.int/gho/en/.)

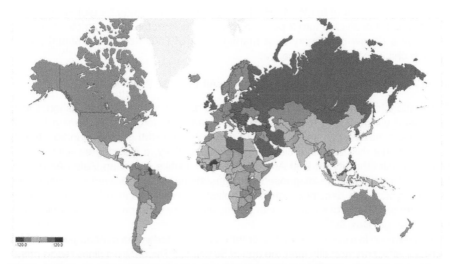

Fig. 5. CVD age-standardized mortality rate, 2012 relative to 2000 (per 100,000). (*Data from* World Health Organization; available at: http://www.who.int/gho/en/.)

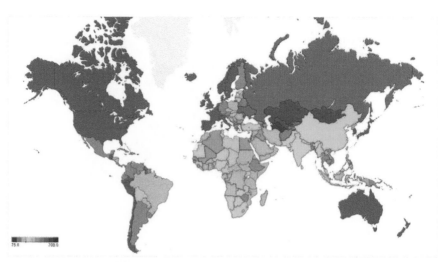

Fig. 6. 2012: Age-standardized CVD mortality rate by country (per 100,000). (*Data from* World Health Organization; available at: http://www.who.int/gho/en/.)

cholesterol-lowering drugs.[41] Investments in health infrastructure and public health programs in developing nations could help alleviate the global burden of CVD.

Smoking remains an important risk for most types of chronic CVD, particularly peripheral arterial disease and abdominal aortic aneurysm. The risk for CVD among smokers remains elevated relative to never-smokers even 10 years after quitting.[42] In a primary care practice, working to optimize patients' risk factor profiles decreases their lifetime risk of CVD.[43] In Western nations, such efforts have led to chronic diseases constituting an increasing portion of initial CVD presentation, including peripheral arterial disease, abdominal aortic aneurysm, heart failure, and stable angina.[34,39]

CLINICAL CORRELATION

CVD is a component of the World Health Organization road map for global NCD. The clinical impact is divided into 2 parts: a review of risk factors and complications followed by a review of primary care management of CVD from the prenatal period through childhood and adolescence.

CLINICAL IMPACT OF SELECT CARDIOVASCULAR DISEASE RISK FACTORS

The relationship between obesity and increased risk of CVD is well-established. DM is associated with a 2-fold to 3-fold increase in artherosclerosis.[44] Screening for DM should be considered in any overweight patient with a BMI greater than 25 (**Box 4**) with additional risk factors, including physical inactivity, a first-degree relative with DM, high-risk ethnicity (African American, Latino, Native American, Asian American, Pacific Islander), women diagnosed with gestational DM or delivering a baby less than 9 pounds, high-density lipoprotein-cholesterol (HDL) less than 35 or triglycerides greater than 250 mg/dL, women with polycystic ovary syndrome, and anyone in the pre-DM range (**Box 5**).[45]

Hypertension is a common risk factor for CVD. Elevated systolic blood pressure has a greater effect on mortality after the age of 50 years.[46] Recent guidelines recommend target blood pressure of lower than 150/90 mm Hg in persons 60 years of age and older and in all other groups, the goal is lower than 140/90 mm Hg.

Box 4	
Obesity classification by body mass index	
Obesity Classification	**BMI**
Underweight	<18.5
Overweight	≥25
Obesity Class I	30.0–34.9
Obesity Class II	35.0–39.9
Obesity Class III	≥40

CKD increases CVD risk and is considered a CVD equivalent. The prevalence of CKD in the United States is roughly 14%.[47] The stage of CKD (**Box 6**), presence of proteinuria, and patient age all affect CVD risk.

COMMUNITY HEALTH

Community-based educational programs using mass media and face-to-face counseling decrease the risk of CVD.[48,49] Social ecological, environmental, and behavioral programs have an impact on community health.[50] Community-based initiatives, such as Healthy People 2020, help reduce health disparities and increase healthy life years by promoting healthy behaviors and enhancing quality of life (**Box 7**).

PREVENTION: THE KEY TO EPIDEMIOLOGIC CHANGE, PRENATAL CARE

Prevention begins before conception. Obesity, DM, and hypertension all have significant implications in pregnancy. Patients should optimize body habitus, normalize any medical issues before pregnancy, and be counseled appropriately. Normal BMI ranges in pregnancy are 18.5 to 24.9 with an anticipated weight gain of 25 to 35 pounds during gestation (http://www.nhlbisupport.com/bmi). Overweight is defined as a BMI of 25 to 29.9; patients in this range should aim for an expected weight gain of 15 to 25 pounds. Obesity in pregnancy is defined as a BMI greater than 30 and has a recommended weight gain of 11 to 20 pounds.[51] In uncomplicated pregnancies, regular physical activity is an important component of health and wellbeing.

It is important to appropriately identify and manage hypertension in all pregnancies. Hypertensive disorders are the second most common cause of maternal death.[52] Hypertensive disorders are categorized as preeclampsia or eclampsia, chronic hypertension, preeclampsia superimposed on chronic hypertension, and gestational hypertension. The diagnosis of hypertension requires 2 abnormal blood pressure readings higher than 140/90. Measurements higher than 160/110 mm Hg are considered severe.

Box 5		
Diabetic diagnostic criteria		
Test	**Pre-DM**	**-DM**
A1C	5.7%–6.4%	>6.5%
FPG	100–125 mg/dL	>126 mg/dL
OGTT	140–199 mg/dL	>200 mg/dL
RPG	—	>200 mg/dL
Abbreviations: A1C, glycosylated hemoglobin percentage; FPG, fasting plasma glucose; OGTT, oral glucose tolerance test; RPG, resting plasma glucose with symptoms of -DM.		

Box 6
Chronic kidney disease stages

Stage 1: Estimated GFR greater than 90 mL/min and persistent proteinuria greater than 3 months

Stage 2: Estimated GFR 60 to 89 mL/min and persistent proteinuria greater than 3 months

Stage 3: Estimated GFR 30 to 59 mL/min

Stage 4: Estimated GFR 15 to 29 mL/min

Stage 5: Estimated GFR less than 15 mL/min and requiring dialysis or transplant

Abbreviation: GFR, glomerular filtration rate.

It is also important to identify congenital cardiac diseases whenever possible (often through the use of antenatal ultrasound). Congenital heart disease affects about 8 out of every 1000 births.[53] There are at least 18 different types of congenital heart disease, many of which can be fixed or repaired through surgery or heart catheterization.[54]

CHILDHOOD AND ADOLESCENCE

After several decades of increasing, the rates of overweight (>85th percentile weight for height) and obesity (>95th percentile weight for height) in American children has stabilized. Family-based and community-based programs promoting physical activity and healthy food decisions have been shown to be effective in reducing childhood obesity.[55] DM has increased in prevalence in children and adolescents. Diabetic patients have a CVD death rate 1.7 times higher than their nondiabetic peers.

PRIMARY PREVENTION IN WOMEN

Heart disease is the leading cause of death in women as well.[56] Misperceptions of CVD as primarily a problem for men and atypical symptoms that are not chest pain contribute to delay in diagnosis (**Box 8**). Risk varies with age of menarche and

---

Box 7
Leading health indicators

- Access to health services
- Clinical preventive services
- Environmental quality
- Injury and violence
- Maternal, infant and child health
- Mental health
- Nutrition, physical activity, and obesity
- Reproductive and sexual health
- Social determinants
- Substance abuse and tobacco

Data from Available at: https://www.healthypeople.gov/.

Box 8
Presentation of heart attack in women

- No symptoms
- Angina pain
- Pain in the jaw, neck, or throat
- Pain in the back
- Pain in the upper abdomen
- Mental stress

---

menopause.[57] Women who experience menopause before the age of 40 years have increased CVD risk.

There are more than 36 million smokers in the United States.[58] Tobacco is the leading cause of preventable death among Americans. The risk of CVD in smokers seems to be dose-related. Atherosclerotic disease progresses more than twice as fast in smokers.[59] Patients with hypertension and DM have even faster disease progression.[60]

Low levels of HDL and high levels of LDL-C are risk factors for developing CVD. Many studies have looked at the effect of cholesterol in the settings of other known risk factors such as hypertension, DM, peripheral vascular disease, smoking, and gender. The Framingham study gave a good estimate on risk stratification in 1998 but was limited to persons of European descent. This was further modified by the Adult Treatment Panel III in 2002, which identified DM as a heart disease equivalent. The Framingham study was reevaluated in 2008 with the Framingham general CVD risk score, which included other atherosclerotic risks such as stroke, peripheral vascular disease, and congestive heart failure. The ACC and AHA have since introduced a model to include race: http://tools.acc.org/ASCVD-Risk-estimator/.

SUMMARY

CVD is a group of disorders of the heart and blood vessels. They present a profound health and economic burden worldwide, accounting for 30% of all global deaths. Of those, 80% are from coronary heart disease and cerebrovascular disease. Wealthy nations have dramatically reduced their CVD burden through coordinated preventive efforts. Poorer nations now represent 75% of the premature mortality from CVD.

Prevention is the best treatment of CVD. Improved preventive measures have led to a 30% decrease in CVD risk in the Western world. Primary care providers are in an ideal position to help patients address their modifiable risk factors for CVD. Most primary preventive efforts target reductions in untreated hypertension, smoking, and sedentary lifestyle. However, ideal preventive measures start in the prenatal period.

Low education, income, and poverty status are barriers to reducing CVD risk. Building health care infrastructure in poorer nations requires addressing those maybe modifiable risk factors. The Global Hearts initiative is a collaborative effort between the World Health Organization, the United States Centers for Disease Control and Prevention, the World Heart Federation, the World Stroke Organization, the International Society of Hypertension, and the World Hypertension League that seeks to reduce CVD risk worldwide. This initiative will use cost-effective interventions at the community and national levels to reduce the CVD burden in poorer nations.

REFERENCES

1. Jousilahti P, Vartiainen E, Tuomilehto J, et al. Sex, age, cardiovascular risk factors, and coronary heart disease: a prospective follow-up study of 14 786 middle-aged men and women in Finland. Circulation 1999;99:1165–72.

2. Kochanek KD, Xu JQ, Murphy SL, et al. Deaths: final data for 2009. Natl Vital Stat Rep 2011;60(3):1–116.

3. Mozaffarian D, Benjamin EJ, Go AS, et al. Heart disease and stroke statistics—2015 update: a report from the American Heart Association. Circulation 2015; 131:e29–322.

4. Lloyd-Jones DM, Nam BH, D'Agostino RB Sr, et al. Parental cardiovascular disease as a risk factor for cardiovascular disease in middle-age adults: a prospective study of parents and offspring. JAMA 2004;291(18):2204–11.

5. Mensah GA, Mokdad AH, Ford ES, et al. State of disparities in cardiovascular health in the United States. Circulation 2005;111(10):1233–41.

6. Lloyd-Jones DM, Leip EP, Larson MG, et al. Prediction of lifetime risk for cardiovascular disease by risk factor burden at 50 years of age. Circulation 2006; 113(6):791–8.

7. Law MR, Wald NJ. Environmental tobacco smoke and ischemic heart disease. Prog Cardiovasc Dis 2003;46(1):31–8.

8. Thun MJ, Myers DG, Day-Lally C, et al. Age and the exposure-response relationships between cigarette smoking and premature death in cancer prevention study II. In: Burns D, Garfinkel L, Samet J, editors. Changes in cigarette-related disease risks and their implications for prevention and control. Smoking and tobacco control monograph No 8. Bethesda (MD): U.S. Department of Health and Human Services, National Cancer Institute; 1997. p. 383–475. NIH Pub No. 97-4213.

9. Dunbar A, Gotsis W, Frishman W. Second-hand tobacco smoke and cardiovascular disease risk: an epidemiological review. Cardiol Rev 2013;21(2):94–100.

10. Wilson PW, D'Agostino RB, Sullivan L, et al. Overweight and obesity as determinants of cardiovascular risk: the Framingham experience. Arch Intern Med 2002; 162(16):1867–72.

11. Poirier P, Giles TD, Bray GA, et al. Obesity and cardiovascular disease: pathophysiology, evaluation, and effect of weight loss. Circulation 2006;113:898–918.

12. Roberson LL, Aneni EC, Maziak W, et al. Beyond BMI: the "metabolically healthy obese" phenotype and its association with clinical and subclinical cardiovascular disease and all-cause mortality, a systematic review. BMC Public Health 2014;14:14.

13. Reddigan JI, Ardern CI, Riddell MC, et al. Relation of physical activity to cardiovascular disease mortality and the influence of cardiometabolic risk factors. Am J Cardiol 2011;108(10):1426–31.

14. Sattelmair J, Pertman J, Ding EL, et al. Dose response between physical activity and risk of coronary heart disease: a meta-analysis. Circulation 2011;124(7): 789–95.

15. Mozaffarian D. Dietary and policy priorities for cardiovascular disease, diabetes, and obesity. Circulation 2016;133(2):187–225.

16. American Heart Association. Alcohol & heart health. 2017. Available at: http://www. heart.org/HEARTORG/HealthyLiving/HealthyEating/Nutrition/Alcohol-and-Heart-Health_UCM_305173_Article.jsp#.WGZ-RHmQyJA. Accessed April 1, 2017.

17. Emberson JR, Bennett DA. Effect of alcohol on risk of coronary heart disease and stroke: causality, bias, or a bit of both? Vasc Health Risk Manag 2006;2(3): 239–49.
18. Kannel WB. Hypertension: reflections on risks and prognostication. Med Clin North Am 2009;93(3):541–58.
19. James PA, Oparil S, Carter BL, et al. 2014 evidence-based guideline for the management of high blood pressure in adults. Report form the panel members appointed to the eight joint national committee (JNC8). JAMA 2014;311(5):507–20.
20. Martín-Timón I, Sevillano-Collantes C, Seguar-Galindo A, et al. Type 2 diabetes and cardiovascular disease: have all risk factors the same strength? World J Diabetes 2014;5(4):440–70.
21. Goff DC, Lloyd-Jones DM, Bennett G, et al. 2013 ACC/AHA guideline on the assessment of cardiovascular risk. Circulation 2014;129:S49–73.
22. Stone NJ, Robinson AH, Lichtenstein CN, et al. 2013 ACC/AHA guideline on the treatment of blood cholesterol to reduce atherosclerotic cardiovascular risk in adults: a report of the American College of Cardiology/American Heart Association Task Force on Practice Guidelines. Circulation 2014;129:S1–45.
23. Steptoe A, Kivimäki M. Stress and cardiovascular disease. Nat Rev Cardiol 2012; 9(6):360–70.
24. Dimsdale JE. Psychological stress and cardiovascular disease. J Am Coll Cardiol 2008;51(13):1237–46.
25. Kassebaum NJ, Arora M, Barber RM, et al. Global, regional, and national disability-adjusted life-years (DALYs) for 315 diseases and injuries and healthy life expectancy (HALE), 1990-2015: a systematic analysis for the Global Burden of Disease Study 2015. Lancet 2016;388(10053):1603–58.
26. Raskob GE, Angchaisuksiri P, Blanco AN, et al. Thrombosis: a major contributor to global disease burden. Thromb Res 2014;134(5):931–8.
27. Townsend N, Nichols M, Scarborough P, et al. Cardiovascular disease in Europe–epidemiological update 2015. Eur Heart J 2015;36(40):2696–705.
28. Mensah GA, Roth GA, Sampson UK, et al. Mortality from cardiovascular diseases in sub-Saharan Africa, 1990-2013: a systematic analysis of data from the Global Burden of Disease Study 2013. Cardiovasc J Afr 2015;26(2 Suppl 1):S6–10.
29. Prabhakaran D, Jeemon P, Roy A. Cardiovascular diseases in India: current epidemiology and future directions. Circulation 2016;133(16):1605–20.
30. Lloyd-Jones DM, Larson MG, Beiser A, et al. Lifetime risk of developing coronary heart disease. Lancet 1999;353:89.
31. Lloyd-Jones DM, Wilson PW, Larson MG, et al. Framingham risk score and prediction of lifetime risk for coronary heart disease. Am J Cardiol 2004;94(1):20–4.
32. Schmidt M, Jacobsen JB, Lash TL, et al. 25 year trends in first time hospitalisation for acute myocardial infarction, subsequent short and long term mortality, and the prognostic impact of sex and comorbidity: a Danish nationwide cohort study. BMJ 2012;344:e356.
33. Koton S, Schneider AL, Rosamond WD, et al. Stroke incidence and mortality trends in US communities, 1987 to 2011. JAMA 2014;312:259.
34. George J, Rapsomaniki E, Pujades-Rodriguez M, et al. How does cardiovascular disease first present in women and men? Incidence of 12 cardiovascular diseases in a contemporary cohort of 1,937,360 people. Circulation 2015; 132:1320.
35. Rapsomaniki E, Timmis A, George J, et al. Blood pressure and incidence of twelve cardiovascular diseases: lifetime risks, healthy life-years lost, and age-specific associations in 1·25 million people. Lancet 2014;383:1899.

36. Zhou B, Bentham J, Di Cesare M, et al. Worldwide trends in blood pressure from 1975 to 2015: a pooled analysis of 1479 population-based measurement studies with 19.1 million participants. Lancet 2017;389:37–55.

37. Roth GA, Forouzanfar MH, Moran AE, et al. Demographic and epidemiologic drivers of global cardiovascular mortality. N Engl J Med 2015;372(14): 1333–41.

38. Mendoza W, Miranda JJ. Global shifts in cardiovascular disease, the epidemiologic transition, and other contributing factors: toward a new practice of global health cardiology. Cardiol Clin 2017;35(1):1–12.

39. Gupta R, Mohan I, Narula J. Trends in coronary heart disease epidemiology in India. Ann Glob Health 2016;82(2):307–15.

40. Farouzanfar MH, Afshin A, Alexander LT, et al. Global, regional, and national comparative risk assessment of 79 behavioural, environmental and occupational, and metabolic risks or clusters of risks, 1990-2015: a systematic analysis for the Global Burden of Disease Study 2015. Lancet 2016;388(10053): 1659–724.

41. Vos T, Allen C, Arora M, et al. Global, regional, and national incidence, prevalence, and years lived with disability for 310 diseases and injuries, 1990-2015: a systematic analysis for the Global Burden of Disease Study 2015. Lancet 2016;388(10053):1545–602.

42. Pujades-Rodriguez M, George J, Shah AD, et al. Heterogeneous associations between smoking and a wide range of initial presentations of cardiovascular disease in 1937360 people in England: lifetime risks and implications for risk prediction. Int J Epidemiol 2015;44(1):129–41.

43. Berry JD, Dyer A, Cai X, et al. Lifetime risks of cardiovascular disease. N Engl J Med 2012;366:321.

44. Kannel WB, McGee DL. Diabetes and cardiovascular disease: the Framingham Study. JAMA 1979;241(19):2035–8.

45. American Diabetes Association. Statistics about diabetes. Available at: http://diabetes.org/diabetes-basics/statistics/. Accessed March 15, 2017.

46. Taylor BC, Wilt TJ, Welch HG. Impact of diastolic and systolic blood pressure on mortality: implications for the definition of 'normal'. J Gen Intern Med 2011;26(7): 685–90.

47. National Institute of Diabetes and Digestive and Kidney Diseases. Kidney disease statistics for the United States. In: Health statistics. 2016. Available at: https://www.niddk.nih.gov/health-information/health-statistics/Pages/kidney-disease-statistics-united-states.aspx. Accessed April 1, 2017.

48. Farquhar JW, Wood PD, Breitrose H, et al. Community education for cardiovascular health. Lancet 1977;309(8023):1192–5.

49. Brown JP, Clark AM, Dalal H, et al. Patient education in the management of coronary heart disease. Cochrane Database Syst Rev 2011;(12):CD008895.

50. Stokols D. Translating social ecological theory into guidelines for community health promotion. Am J Health Promot 1996;10(4):282–98.

51. American College of Obstetricians and Gynecologists. Weight gain during pregnancy: committee opinion no. 548. Obstet Gynecol 2013;121(1):210–2.

52. Khan KD, Wojdyla D, Say L. WHO analysis of causes of maternal death: a systematic review. Lancet 2006;367(9516):1066–74.

53. National Heart, Lung, and Blood Institute. What are congenital heart defects? Available at: https://www.nhlbi.nih.gov/health/health-topics/topics/chd. Accessed April 1, 2017.

54. American Heart Association. About congenital heart defects. 2017. Available at: http://www.heart.org/HEARTORG/Conditions/CongenitalHeartDefects/About CongenitalHeartDefects/About-Congenital-Heart-Defects_UCM_001217_Article. jsp#.WNhOzIWcHg8. Accessed April 1, 2017.
55. Golan M, Crow S. Targeting parents exclusively in the treatment of childhood obesity: long-term results. Obesity 2004;12(2):357–61.
56. Douglas PS, Daubert MA. Heart disease in women. Circulation 2016;133:e5–6.
57. Canoy D, Beral V, Balkwill A, et al. Age at menarche and risks of coronary heart and other vascular diseases in a large UK cohort. Circulation 2015;131(3): 237–44.
58. Center for Disease Control. Smoking and tobacco use. In: Data and statistics: fast facts and fact sheets. 2017. Available at: https://www.cdc.gov/tobacco/ data_statistics/fact_sheets/. Accessed April 1, 2017.
59. Howard G, Wagenknecht LE, Burke GL, et al. The Atherosclerosis Risk in Communities (ARIC) study. JAMA 1998;279(2):119–24.
60. U.S. Department of Health and Human Services. E-cigarette use among youth and young adults: a report of the surgeon general. 2015. Available at: https://e-cigarettes.surgeongeneral.gov/documents/2016_SGR_Fact_Sheet_508.pdf. Accessed April 1, 2017.

Heavy Heart
The Economic Burden of Heart Disease in the United States Now and in the Future

Andrew J. Foy, MD[a],*, John M. Mandrola, MD[b]

KEYWORDS

- Health care costs • Cardiovascular care • Health economics • Overuse

KEY POINTS

- Cardiovascular disease represents a significant financial burden to the US population.
- Based on current trends, spending on cardiovascular disease will continue to increase significantly in the upcoming years.
- A substantial portion of cardiovascular care that is currently provided confers little clinical efficacy over less expensive alternatives, and some practices may be unnecessary.
- Physicians can limit unnecessary spending by avoiding flat-of-the-curve practices and optimizing the use of tests and procedures.

The United States spends more on health care than any other industrialized nation. In 2016, health care expenditure reached an estimated $3.35 trillion or $10,345 per individual.[1]

Cardiovascular disease (CVD) represents the leading cause of death and disability as well as the most significant source of health care spending. This article reviews the current economic burden of heart disease in the United States, presents future projections, and explores factors driving cost growth in cardiovascular care.

THE COST OF CARDIOVASCULAR CARE AND FUTURE PROJECTIONS

Approximately 82.6 million American adults (1 of every 3) have some form of CVD.[2] The most common is hypertension (76.4 million) followed by coronary heart disease (CHD) (16.3 million), stroke (7 million), and congestive heart failure (CHF) (5.7 million).[2] The prevalence and incidence rates of these conditions vary by age, sex, and race/ethnicity.[3,4]

Disclosure Statement: The authors have nothing to disclose.
[a] Cardiology Division, Penn State College of Medicine, 500 University Drive, PO Box 850 H047, Hershey, PA 17078, USA; [b] Louisville Cardiology Group at Baptist Health, 3900 Kresge Way, Suite 60, Louisville, KY 40207, USA
* Corresponding author.
E-mail address: afoy@hmc.psu.edu

Prim Care Clin Office Pract 45 (2018) 17–24
https://doi.org/10.1016/j.pop.2017.11.002   primarycare.theclinics.com
0095-4543/18/© 2017 Elsevier Inc. All rights reserved.

The incidence of symptomatic CHD, defined as having angina or a heart attack, is rare in men before the age of 45, occurring in only 1 out of every 333 but affects 1 out of 14 men older than 85.[2] Women have similar rates of CHD compared with men, but they occur 10 years later in life. Women also have a higher proportion of CVD events due to stroke.[2] Men have a 52% risk for developing CVD over a lifetime compared with 39% for women. The overall survival rate following the development of some form of CVD is 30 years for men and 36 years for women.[5]

The costs of cardiovascular care impose a significant burden on the US health care system. The American Heart Association estimated that in 2006, the cost of CVD (including CHD, stroke, hypertensive heart disease, and CHF) was $457 billion.[6] The *direct cost* to payers for hospitalizations, physician visits, pharmaceuticals, and rehabilitation services was estimated at $292 billion with the remainder accounted for by indirect costs due to productivity losses from premature mortality and morbidity.[6] As a point of comparison, spending on CVD in 2006 was equal to more than half of what the US government (federal, state, and local) spent on education ($812 billion); more than two-thirds of what it spent on defense ($622 billion); and more than what was spent on welfare ($320 billion) and transportation ($229 billion).[7]

An aging population and increase in chronic disease are expected to further increase the cost of CVD in the United States over the next 20 years.[8] It is estimated that between 2010 and 2030, the cost of CVD in the United States will increase to more than $1 trillion (in 2008 dollars).[8] Total direct and indirect costs will increase from $273 billion to $818 billion and $172 to $276 billion, respectively.

IMPLICATIONS FOR INDIVIDUALS AND THE HEALTH CARE SYSTEM

Massive increases in health care spending (CVD, in particular) are likely to be favorable for the medical industry in the United States. These increases, however, will likely have negative consequences for individuals and the general population. To accommodate increased spending, health insurance premiums will continue to increase in the private sector and may accelerate disproportionately. To date, premium increases have had a negative impact on workers, contributing to wage stagnation and social unrest.

The primary reason for wage stagnation over the last several decades relates to the rising costs of health insurance benefits. The Kaiser Family Foundation reported that between 1999 and 2011, health insurance premiums increased 168%, whereas (over the same period) total earnings increased by only 50%.[9] This divergence in health insurance premiums and earnings has been termed the *affordability gap*. According to a report of 487 US employers with at least 1000 employees, the total cost of health insurance per employee (counting both the employer and the employee contribution) increased from $9748 in 2009 to $12,041 in 2015.[10]

Increased health care spending also threatens government programs like Medicare and Medicaid. Medicare is federally funded. Currently, less than half of its spending derives from payroll taxes. The majority comes from general revenue transfers and another minority from premiums. Medicare spending has far exceeded its originally intended revenue source of payroll taxes, requiring ever-increasing premiums and general revenue transfers to maintain solvency (**Fig. 1**).[11]

At the state level, Medicaid faces even greater challenges. Unlike the federal government, state governments cannot run deficits (aided by monetary policy) with the ability to borrow at artificially low interest rates. Thus, states facing economic challenges must limit Medicaid costs by reducing payments. Reduced payments further limits available options for the most vulnerable patients, many of whom suffer from CVD-related conditions.

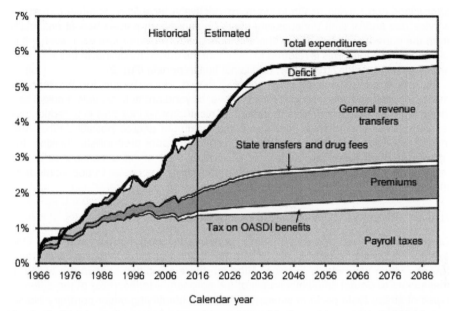

Fig. 1. Medicare spending sources over time. OASDI, old age, survivors, and disability insurance. *From* The Boards of Trustees, Federal Hospital Insurance and Federal Supplementary Medical Insurance Trust Funds. The 2017 Annual Report of the Boards of Trustees of the Federal Hospital Insurance and Federal Supplementary Medical Insurance Trust Funds. Available at: https://www.cms.gov/Research-Statistics-Data-and-Systems/Statistics-Trends-and-Reports/ReportsTrustFunds/Downloads/TR2017.pdf. Accessed October 12, 2017.

EXPLORING COST GROWTH IN CARDIOVASCULAR CARE

It is difficult to understand or appreciate cost growth in cardiovascular care without understanding overall trends in US health care spending. Several factors contribute to the escalating spending trajectory: (1) an aging population with increasing comorbidities; (2) technological advances in health care; (3) supply-induced (flat-of-the-curve) medical care and resultant medical overuse.

From 1970 to 2014, life expectancy at birth increased about 10 years in men (from 67 to 77) and by 5 years in women (from 75 to 80).[12] Over the same period (taking into account general inflation), health care spending per individual increased by more than 500%, rising from $1714 to $9255 per person per year.[13] This increase in health care spending markedly exceeds gains in life expectancy.

Direct spending on medical care plays a small role in population health and cardiovascular health. Although the exact percentages are debatable, it is generally thought that clinical care contributes only about 10% toward population health and premature death. Given this as a background, why do Americans spend so much on medical care (in general) and cardiovascular care (in particular)? To help answer this, it is important to illustrate how the current system is perfectly designed to deliver the results it achieves.

In the United States, fee for service is the predominant reimbursement model for medical care rendered to patients. Most care is paid for by a third party (eg, health insurance company), which is privately administered and accountable to shareholders. This creates a situation wherein those who provide and pay for medical care (physicians and private health insurers, respectively) have little incentive to restrain service use and/or limit unnecessary costs because both parties benefit financially from the current structure. Thus, there is incentive to provide more care, even if it is of uncertain benefit. This is referred to as "flat of the curve" medicine. In this situation, additional care yields little, if any, additional health benefit (**Fig. 2**).

Flat-of-the-curve medical care is "supply-induced," driven by supply rather than demand. Physicians have an additional incentive, beyond profit, to provide medical services that offer little to no value to patients. This additional incentive is to reduce risk (to themselves and to their patients) to the maximum degree possible. When this incentive toward "defensive medicine" is paired with poor probabilistic thinking, the "more-is-better" American culture, profit motive, lack of price transparency, and removal of direct checks and balances on spending, it is easier to appreciate how the current system often promotes flat-of-the-curve medical care.

FLAT OF THE CURVE CARE IN CARDIOVASCULAR MEDICINE

Cardiovascular medicine has multiple potential flat-of-the-curve practices. One example is cardiac stress testing. There are many forms of cardiovascular stress testing, which vary widely in price. Although there are differences in the ability of these tests to detect small blockages of the coronary arteries, most of the different types of stress tests perform similarly in terms of identifying major coronary blockages. In terms of patient-centered outcomes, no single test has consistently been found to be superior to the others. In a normal market, the cheapest test would be the most common test chosen. In terms of stress testing, one source reveals that a nuclear stress test provided "in-network" in central Pennsylvania costs 15-fold more than a graded exercise electrocardiography (ECG) test.[14] Despite a large difference in costs between these 2 tests (which yield remarkably similar results in terms of outcomes that matter most to patients), exercise ECG tests are ordered much less frequently than their more expensive counterparts. Another study of privately insured patients seen in emergency departments across the country for

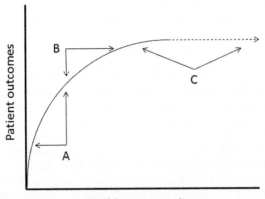

Health care spending

Fig. 2. Schematic representation of flat-of-the-curve medicine. At point A, additional health care spending is associated with significant improvement in patient outcomes. At point B, additional health care spending remains associated with improvement in patient outcomes, but the yield or effectiveness of the additional spending on patient outcomes is diminished compared with point A. At point C, additional spending is not associated with significant improvement in patient outcomes. Point C is what is referred to as "flat of the curve."

chest pain similarly showed that nuclear stress tests were ordered more frequently than exercise ECG tests (65% vs 14%).[15]

Drug-eluting stents (DES) represent another common flat-of-the-curve practice in cardiovascular medicine. More than 1 million patients undergo coronary artery stenting each year in the United States. Stenting procedures using bare-metal stents (BMS) confer a significant advantage for maintaining vessel patency following balloon angioplasty. A patient-centered, clinically meaningful advantage for DES over BMS has never been demonstrated. A large, randomized controlled clinical trial, The Norwegian Coronary Stent Trial, found no advantage for DES over BMS in terms of reducing death or nonfatal myocardial infarction over 5 years of follow-up.[16] Furthermore, there was no difference in quality-of-life measures between the 2 groups.[16] In the United States, the average price of DES exceeds $1500 compared with $700 for BMS.[17] Additional costs of DES include the need for extended dual-antiplatelet therapy and the associated increase in bleeding risk. Despite the increase in cost and lack of clinical superiority, DES are used more commonly. Targeted marketing, the use of surrogate endpoints, and the use of data from (potentially biased) industry-sponsored clinical trials may contribute to these differences in practice.

FLAT-OF-THE-CURVE "EXPANDED USE" IN CARDIOVASCULAR MEDICINE

In the preceding section, nuclear stress testing was presented as an example of a flat-of-the-curve practice compared with exercise ECG. Interestingly, cardiac stress testing of any kind has never been found to reduce heart attacks or help people live longer.[18] The main use of stress testing is to identify the likely cause of chest-pain symptoms, risk stratify, and improve quality of life in patients with chest discomfort due to a major coronary occlusion. When blockages are identified, specific treatments can be provided to improve or relieve the discomfort and improve quality of life.

Over the last several decades, the use of stress testing (in particular, nuclear stress testing) has increased considerably in the United States. The percentage of stress tests with evidence of ischemia has declined, however, from 30% to 5%.[19] This reduction in positive test results reflects an expansion in overall use, as opposed to an increase in use for similar at-risk patients. If the latter occurred, it could be inferred that stress testing was previously underused and that the increased use conferred an advantage to the population. In such a case, an increase in use would not be accompanied by a significant decline in test positivity. However, increased use in the setting of an associated reduction in test positivity suggests expansion of stress testing to patients who may not be good candidates for the test in terms of pretest disease probability.

A report on temporal trends in the use of common diagnostic tests and treatments for CVD in the United States between 1993 and 2001 among Medicare fee-for-service patients[20] highlights flat-of-the-curve expansion for the use of stress testing, cardiac catheterization, and revascularization. Rates for each nearly doubled over an 8-year period, from 56.1 to 102.2/1000; 21.9 to 37.0/1000; 10.9 to 18.2/1000. During this same time, however, the rate of acute myocardial infarction was unchanged (8.6–8.7/1000) (**Fig. 3**).[20]

SUPPLY-SENSITIVE CARDIOVASCULAR CARE

Cost containment is an active point of conversation in current US health care delivery debate. One way to reduce medical costs is to identify and reduce (or eliminate) the

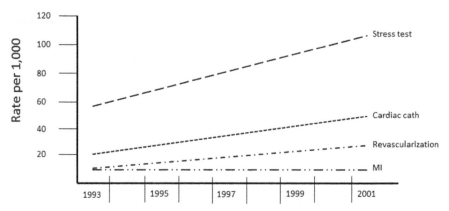

Fig. 3. Flat-of-the-curve expansion of common cardiac tests and treatments. cath, catheterization; MI, myocardial infarction.

use of unnecessary procedures or care processes. Proving that a test or procedure is unnecessary, however, is very difficult. Head-to-head trials may not be possible for financial, ethical, and/or practical reasons. The provision of unnecessary care, therefore, must sometimes be inferred from studies that show a significant variation in practice without notable differences in relevant health outcomes. Flat-of-the-curve practices in cardiovascular medicine may help illustrate this trend in supply-sensitive care. As one example, large variations in practices from state to state, county to county, hospital to hospital, and physician to physician not associated with differences in health outcomes suggest that use of a particular service is unnecessary. Often the most significant factor associated with an increase in utilization is access.

To illustrate this point, examine one study comparing the use of stress testing in different hospitals across the United States.[21] In this particular study of patients presenting to the emergency department with chest pain but no myocardial infarction, practices varied dramatically from hospital to hospital. Hospitals in the lowest quartile of use performed stress testing in 6% of patients, whereas those in the highest quartile performed stress testing on 35% of patients. Hospitals in the highest quartile were nearly 5 times more likely to subsequently perform invasive angiography and 4 times more likely to perform coronary revascularization procedures compared with facilities with lower use of stress tests. Despite these large differences in stress testing, patient-centered outcomes (eg, readmission for myocardial infarction) did not differ between groups. The factor most highly related to stress test utilization was access to the procedure.

The volume of procedures differs widely by geography as well. In another study of elderly patients with acute myocardial infarction,[22] cardiac procedures in the United States far exceeded those in Canada. Despite this, the decline in 1-year mortality was unchanged, and there was no difference in rehospitalization for myocardial infarction between groups. Notably, however, there was a much higher density of cardiac catheterization laboratories in the United States. A similar comparison of trends in cardiac procedures between New York State and Ontario, Canada[23] showed that for non-acute indications, the age- and sex-adjusted rate of coronary artery stenting was 2.3 times higher in New York. This was also associated with a higher density of interventional facilities, which was thought to be at least partially attributable to the market-oriented financing approach in New York.

SUMMARY

CVD represents a significant financial burden to the US population. Based on current trends, spending on CVD will continue to increase significantly in the upcoming years. Despite being a leading cause of death and disability, a substantial portion of cardiovascular care that is currently provided confers little clinical efficacy over less expensive alternatives, and some practices may be unnecessary. Continued growth in health care spending limits spending in other areas, and although physicians may not be able to directly change health policy, they can limit unnecessary spending by avoiding flat-of-the-curve practices and optimizing the use of tests and procedures.

REFERENCES

1. Keehan SP, Poisal JA, Cuckler GA, et al. National health expenditure projections, 2015-25: economy, prices, and aging expected to shape spending and enrollment. Health Aff 2016;35:1522–31.
2. Roger V, Go A, Lloyd-Jones DM, et al. Heart disease and stroke statistics – 2011 update: a report from the American Heart Association. Circulation 2011;123: e18–209.
3. Pleis JR, Ward BW, Lucas JW. Summary health statistics for U.S. adults: National Health Interview Survey, 2009. Vital Health Stat 2010;(249):1–207. Available at: http://www.cdc.gov/nchs/data/series/sr_10/sr10_249.pdf. Accessed April 10, 2017.
4. National Institutes of Health, National Heart, Lung, and Blood Institute. Incidence and prevalence: 2006 chart book on cardiovascular and lung diseases. Bethesda (MD): National Heart, Lung, and Blood Institute; 2006. Available at: http://www.nhlbi.nih.gov/resources/docs/06a_ip_chtbk.pdf. Accessed April 10, 2017.
5. Lloyd-Jones DM, Leip EP, Larson MG, et al. Prediction of lifetime risk for cardiovascular disease by risk factor burden at 50 years of age. Circulation 2006;113:791–8.
6. Thom T, Haase N, Rosamond W, et al. Heart disease and stroke statistics – 2006 update: a report from the American Heart Association Statistics Committee and Stroke Statistics Subcommittee. Circulation 2006;113:e85–151.
7. US Government Spending 2016. Available at: http://www.usgovernmentspending. com/year2016_0.html. Accessed March 9, 2017.
8. Heidenreich PA, Trogdon JG, Khavjou OA, et al. Forecasting the future of cardiovascular disease in the United States: a policy statement from the American Heart Association. Circulation 2011;123:933–44.
9. Claxton G, Rae M, Panchal N, et al. Employer health benefits 2011 annual survey. Available at: http://ehbs.kff.org/pdf/2011/8225.pdf. Accessed February 10, 2012.
10. Available at: https://www.thehortongroup.com/sites/default/files/pdf/2652011548 32617.pdf. Accessed April 20, 2017.
11. The Boards of Trustees, Federal Hospital Insurance and Federal Supplementary Medical Insurance Trust Funds. The 2017 Annual Report of the Boards of Trustees of the Federal Hospital Insurance and Federal Supplementary Medical Insurance Trust Funds. Available at: https://www.cms.gov/Research-Statistics-Data-and-Systems/Statistics-Trends-and-Reports/ReportsTrustFunds/Downloads/TR2017.pdf. Accessed October 12, 2017.
12. World Health Organization. Global health observatory (GHO) data. Healthy life expectancy (HALE) at birth. Available at: http://www.who.int/gho/mortality_burden_disease/life_tables/hale/en/. Accessed April 18, 2017.
13. Available at: http://www.healthsystemtracker.org/brief/assessing-the-cost-and-performance-of-the-u-s-health-system/#item-start. Accessed April 18, 2017.

14. Available at: http://www.fairhealthconsumer.org. Accessed October 10, 2017.
15. Foy AJ, Liu G, Davidson WR Jr, et al. Comparative effectiveness of diagnostic testing strategies in emergency department patients with chest pain. JAMA Intern Med 2015;175:428–36.
16. Bønaa KH, Mannsverk J, Wiseth R, et al. Drug-eluting or bare-metal stents for coronary artery disease. N Engl J Med 2016;375:1242–52.
17. Adams, W. Purchasing insight: coronary artery stents. Available at: https://www.mdbuyline.com/research-library/articles/purchasing-insight-coronary-artery-stents/. Accessed October 10, 2017.
18. Garber AM, Solomon NA. Cost-effectiveness of alternative test strategies for the diagnosis of coronary artery disease. Ann Intern Med 1999;130:719–28.
19. Rozanski A, Gransar H, Hayes SW, et al. Temporal trends in the frequency of inducible myocardial ischemia during cardiac stress testing: 1991 to 2009. J Am Coll Cardiol 2013;61:1054–65.
20. Lucas FL, DeLorenzo MA, Siewers AE, et al. Temporal trends in the utilization of diagnostic testing and treatments for cardiovascular disease in the United States, 1993-2001. Circulation 2006;113:374–9.
21. Safavi KC, Li SX, Dharmarajan K, et al. Hospital variation in the use of noninvasive cardiac imaging and its association with downstream testing, interventions, and outcomes. JAMA Intern Med 2014;174:546–53.
22. Pilote L, Saynina O, Lavoie F, et al. Cardiac procedure use and outcomes in elderly patients with acute myocardial infarction in the United States and Quebec, Canada, 1988 to 1994. Med Care 2003;41:813–22.
23. Ko DT, Tu JV, Samadashvili Z, et al. Temporal trends in the use of percutaneous coronary intervention and coronary artery bypass surgery in New York state and Ontario. Circulation 2010;121:2635–44.

Prevention of Cardiovascular Disease

Brian V. Reamy, MD[a],*, Pamela M. Williams, MD[b,c],
Daniel P. Kuckel, MD, MS, MBA[d]

KEYWORDS

- Cardiovascular disease prevention • Risk assessment for cardiovascular disease
- Diets for cardiovascular disease prevention • Life's Simple 7

KEY POINTS

- 90% of cardiovascular disease (CVD) events can be prevented.
- A formal 10-year and lifetime CVD risk assessment should be performed using a global risk calculator.
- Each patient should have an individualized CVD prevention prescription grounded in the American Heart Association Simple 7.
- The patients at the highest risk should have the most intensive prevention interventions.
- Life's Simple 7 include: tobacco avoidance, regular exercise, normal BMI, healthy diet, ideal lipids, ideal glucose, and blood pressure.

INTRODUCTION

Despite decades of significant advances in understanding the pathophysiology and risk factors that contribute to heart disease and stroke, cardiovascular disease (CVD) remains the leading cause of death in the United States and worldwide. One of every three deaths in the United States is from CVD. It kills more people than all forms of cancer and respiratory diseases combined and is the primary killer of women.[1]

Disclosure Statement: All authors are Federal Employees and have nothing to disclose. The article represents the views of the authors and not the views of the Uniformed Services University, the Department of the Air Force, the Department of the Navy, or the Department of Defense.
[a] F. Edward Hebert School of Medicine, Uniformed Services University, Office of the Senior Associate Dean for Academic and Faculty Affairs, 4301 Jones Bridge Road, Bethesda, MD 20814, USA; [b] Mike O'Callaghan Federal Medical Center, 99MDG/DME, 4700 Las Vegas Boulevard North, Nellis AFB, NV 89191, USA; [c] F. Edward Hebert School of Medicine, Uniformed Services University, Bethesda, MD, USA; [d] Naval Hospital Jacksonville, 2080 Child Street, Jacksonville, FL 32214, USA
* Corresponding author.
E-mail address: brian.reamy@usuhs.edu

Yet, prevention of CVD is an achievable goal. A rigorous 2010 analysis by the World Health Organization demonstrated that reducing risk factors in young adults and maintaining an optimum risk profile through age 50 could prevent 90% of atherosclerotic CVD events.[2] Unfortunately, data from the National Health and Nutrition Examination Survey indicate that only 1% of the US population maintains such an ideal risk profile into adulthood.[3]

The reasons for this are many, ranging from misinformation and poor implementation of proven preventive strategies by physicians, to patients' misplaced fears of medications or incorrect understanding of ideal dietary and lifestyle choices. Each patient should have an individualized "prescription" for CVD prevention that incorporates modalities to control the seven modifiable cardiovascular risk factors:

1. Tobacco cessation
2. Weight management
3. Physical activity
4. Diet
5. Blood cholesterol
6. Blood glucose
7. Blood pressure

Preventive prescriptions can be viewed as primary, secondary, or primordial.

PRIMARY, SECONDARY, AND PRIMORDIAL PREVENTION

Primary prevention is the prevention of CVD before the onset of any clinical manifestations of disease. Primary prevention assesses individualized risk for disease and targets preventive efforts to reduce clinical events. Secondary prevention is the prevention of recurrent disease after an initial clinical event. Secondary prevention optimizes risk factors and aims to reverse existing CVD.

Primordial prevention involves the early establishment of habits and lifestyle choices that prevent the development of CVD risk factors. Ideally primordial prevention starts in utero, continues through infancy, childhood, adolescence, and into young adulthood through tobacco avoidance, daily activity, healthy diet, and weight management.

RISK ASSESSMENT AND THE USE OF GLOBAL RISK CALCULATORS

Calculating an individual patient's risk for CVD guides the type and intensity of preventive interventions. Currently there are no internationally agreed on guidelines for risk assessment and subsequent interventions.[4] Most guidelines incorporate age, sex, smoking, blood pressure, lipid levels, family history of premature CVD, and ethnicity. Multiple calculators to determine 10-year absolute risk for CVD have been developed and studied internationally. Those currently in use include the American College of Cardiology (ACC)/American Heart Association (AHA) Pooled Cohort Risk Assessment (United States; http://www.cvriskcalculator.com/), the National Vascular Disease Prevention Alliance (Australia; http://www.cvdcheck. org.au), and the QRISK2-2016 score (United Kingdom; https://qrisk.org/2016/). These risk calculators provide lifetime risk calculations and estimations of risk reduction if preventive interventions are successfully implemented. The ACC/ AHA Pooled Cohort equation is the only US CVD risk prediction model with external validation.[5] **Table 1** compares and contrasts results and recommendations from three different risk calculators: (1) Australia's National Vascular Disease Prevention Alliance, (2) UK National Institute for Health and Care Excellence QRISK score, and (3) the ACC/AHA 10-year Pooled Cohort Risk Assessment, in a

Table 1
Comparison of global risk calculators

	National Vascular Disease Prevention Alliance (Australia)	QRISK 2 (United Kingdom)	ACC/AHA (United States)
Shared variables (among all three calculators)	Age 50 Gender male SBP 140 mm Hg Smoking status + Tchol 200 mg/dL HDL 40 mg/dL Diabetes –	Age (24–84) 50 Gender male SBP 140 mm Hg Smoking status + Diabetes - Cholesterol/HDL ratio 5	Age 50 Gender male SBP 140 mm Hg Smoking status + Tchol 200 mg/dL HDL mg/dL Diabetes –

Unique variables	Echocardiogram demonstrating left ventricular hypertrophy (–)	Ethnicity (white)
		UK postal code (blank)
		Angina/CVD first-
		  degree relative (–)
		CKD stage 4/5 (–)
		Hypertension
		  medication (–)
		RA (–)
		BMI 25
			Race (white)
			DBP 85 mm Hg
			Hypertension
			  medication (–)

10-y risk score	12% (no statin recommended)	9.6% (no statin recommended)	11.2% (statin use recommended)

Data calculated using available online tools demonstrating a comparison among three different risk calculators in a hypothetical 50-year-old white male with BMI 25, smoker, total cholesterol of 200 and HDL of 40 mg/dL, blood pressure 140/85 mm Hg, and no other comorbidities. Each calculator demonstrated elevated 10-year risk but only the ACC/AHA calculator recommended statin use (moderate to high intensity).

Abbreviations: BMI, body mass index; CKD, chronic kidney disease; HDL, high-density lipoprotein; RA, Rheumatoid Arthritis; SBP, systolic blood pressure; Tchol, total cholesterol.

Data from Refs.[4,6–8]

hypothetical 50-year-old white man with body mass index (BMI) of 25, smoker, total cholesterol of 200 mg/dL, and a high-density lipoprotein (HDL) of 40 mg/dL. The US Preventive Services Task Force makes no recommendation for, or against, lipid screening in young adults without Coronary Heart Disease risk factors.[6]

CARDIOVASCULAR DISEASE PREVENTION AND THE SIMPLE 7

In 2010, the AHA established a 2020 impact goal of improving the cardiovascular health of all Americans by 20%, while reducing deaths from CVD and stroke by 20%.[9] To achieve this goal, the AHA developed an updated strategy emphasizing the benefits of healthy living as foundational to increasing the chance of living free of CVD, and to reduce the burden of disease. Targeting preventive efforts against smoking, physical inactivity, elevated blood cholesterol, uncontrolled high blood pressure, obesity, and diabetes has reduced mortality from coronary heart disease by 31% and stroke mortality by 29%.[9] Although there was also a reduction in the prevalence of uncontrolled blood pressure, high cholesterol, and smoking, the prevalence of obesity and diabetes increased and that of physical inactivity remained largely unchanged.[9] Emphasizing healthy lifestyle behaviors is also a key focus in international guidelines.[10–12]

The inverse relationship between ideal cardiovascular health and CVD incidence is well-established.[13] The association between ideal cardiovascular health and reductions in non-CVD is also becoming increasingly clear.[14,15] Thus, a cardiovascular risk prevention strategy that comprehensively applies these Simple 7 metrics to all patients in an integrated manner is an effective framework for clinical efforts in the primordial, primary, and secondary prevention of CVD.

Based on evidence from randomized clinical trials and epidemiologic studies, the AHA identified seven ideal cardiovascular health metrics, Life's Simple 7 (**Table 2**), which encompass four ideal health behaviors (nonsmoking, BMI <25 kg/m^2, physical activity at goal levels, and diet consistent with recommended guidelines) and three ideal health factors (untreated total cholesterol <200 mg/dL, blood pressure <120/80 mm Hg, and fasting blood glucose <100 mg/dL).[9] Although the health-promoting benefits of each health behavior and health factor have been individually established, the definition of ideal cardiovascular health requires an individual to meet all seven components. Few global citizens meet all seven cardiovascular health metrics.[14]

Table 2
Definition of ideal cardiovascular health

Goal/Metric	Ideal Cardiovascular Health Definition
Current smoking	
Adults >20 y of age	Never or quit >12 mo ago
Children 12–19 y of age	Never tried; never smoked whole cigarette
Body mass index	
Adults >20 y of age	<25 kg/m^2
Children 2–19 y of age	<85th percentile
Physical activity	
Adults >20 y of age	≥150 min/wk moderate intensity or ≥75 min/wk vigorous intensity or combination
Children 12–19 y of age	≥60 min of moderate- or vigorous-intensity activity every day
Healthy diet score[a]	
Adults >20 y of age	4–5 components[a]
Children 5–19 y of age	4–5 components[a]
Total cholesterol	
Adults >20 y of age	<200 mg/dL[b]
Children 6–19 y of age	<170 mg/dL[b]
Blood pressure	
Adults >20 y of age	<120/<80 mm Hg[b]
Children 8–19 y of age	<90th percentile[b]
Fasting plasma glucose	
Adults >20 y of age	<100 mg/dL[b]
Children 12–19 y of age	<100 mg/dL[b]

[a] The committee selected five aspects of diet to define a healthy dietary score. The score is not intended to be comprehensive. Rather, it is a practical approach that provides individuals with a set of potential concrete actions. A comprehensive rationale is set forth in the text of this document, and a comprehensive set of nutrition recommendations is provided in the 2006 Nutrition Guidelines.
[b] Untreated values.
From Lloyd-Jones DM, Hong Y, Labarthe D, et al. Defining and setting national goals for cardiovascular health promotion and disease reduction: the American Heart Association's strategic impact goal through 2020 and beyond. Circulation 2010;121:591; with permission.

A CLOSER LOOK AT THE SIMPLE 7: TOBACCO CESSATION

Smoking is a significant risk factor for CVD that should be assessed and addressed at every clinical encounter.[16] Two techniques are effective in promoting smoking cessation: motivational interviewing (MI) and the 5 A's Framework (ask, advise, assess, assist, arrange).[17,18] MI is a counseling method that engages a patient's intrinsic motivation to make a positive behavioral changes to improve health. MI includes an assessment of a patient's readiness to change: precontemplation (no intention to quit), contemplation (considering change within the next 6 months), preparation (planning to take action within the next month), action (actively changing), and maintenance (greater than 6 months since behavior change).[16,18] Patients are asked how important the given change is to them and how confident they are to make the needed behavioral change.

The 5 A's Framework includes adding smoking as a vital sign to all patients' charts (Asking), offering clear support for smoking cessation and counseling on its benefits (Advising), discussing willingness and barriers to quitting (Assessing), offering resources for nicotine withdrawal symptoms to include associated depression and weight gain (Assisting), and setting a quit date while committing to a follow-up plan (Arranging).[16,19]

Pharmacotherapy is used as a successful tobacco cessation adjunct. Heavy smokers (those smoking >25 cigarettes/day) should be encouraged to use the patch-plus method in which a slow delivery patch is added to a more rapid acting nicotine-replacement therapy, such as a nicotine gum or lozenge.[16] Bupropion improves smoking cessation rates in some patients compared with placebo and is used with the patch-plus method for additional benefit.[20] Varenicline is another option. Recent data suggest an increased risk of coronary events with varenicline; hence bupropion is recommended if there is concern for CVD.[16,21,22] Clonidine and nortriptyline are traditionally second-line agents that may be helpful, particularly if bupropion or varenicline are contraindicated. Complementary and alternative therapies, such as acupuncture, exercise, and hypnotherapy, may be useful although they lack consistent evidence to support regular use. One notable exception is the use of telephone quit lines, which evidence shows have a several-fold benefit in promoting smoking cessation compared with counseling alone.[16,23]

WEIGHT MANAGEMENT

Most Americans are either overweight (60% of US adults) or obese (30%).[24–26] Unhealthy eating habits combine with inadequate physical activity patterns to explain much of this phenomenon. There are multiple reasons for poor adherence to dietary recommendations; inadequate knowledge, lack of motivation, poor access to healthy foods (food desert), and easy access to unhealthy foods (food swamp) are several examples. Additionally, health care providers are often unfamiliar with dietary guidelines.[24] Currently, the six highest sources of energy in the American diet are burgers and tacos, sweet desserts, sugar-sweetened beverages, rice/pasta, chips/snacks, and pizza.[4,5] As a group these six foods provide 43.2% of the total energy intake in the American diet.[23] Desserts and sugar-sweetened beverages alone provide 15% of the total daily energy intake.[25] Armed with this knowledge, primary care physicians are well-positioned to make an impact in the primary prevention of obesity by counseling patients to avoid these highly processed, energy-dense food products whenever possible.

Weight management is often a difficult conversation for providers and patients alike. Barriers include the lack of knowledge regarding diet and physical activity recommendations for specific medical conditions, lack of core competencies required to perform lifestyle counseling, provider skepticism regarding a patient's willingness to change, and lack of emphasis on physical activity and dietary counseling in medical education. As with tobacco cessation, the cornerstone of effective behavioral counseling is a patient-centered approach using MI and the 5 A's Framework.[27]

An individualized approach to weight management may include the US Department of Agriculture's Daily Food Plans and Super Tracker (www.choosemyplate.gov), MyFitnessPal, Lose It, or applications for use on smart phones.[24] Electronic diaries help achieve a heart-healthy dietary pattern, and a session with a registered dietician is recommended to explain the diary and improve compliance.[24] Goal setting and self-monitoring are important strategies for changing diet and eating behaviors.[24] Goal setting targets specific changes, such as a daily calorie limit or eating breakfast daily. Self-monitoring uses a systematic recording of daily behavior (dietary intake) typically using an electronic tracking tool. Although self-monitoring is challenging to sustain, it can help improve diet and promote weight loss.[24,28,29]

PHYSICAL ACTIVITY

Physical activity is a superb, yet underutilized, prescription for CVD prevention. Any increase in individual physical activity levels is generally associated with a reduced cardiovascular risk. Most adults should aim for 150 minutes of moderate-intensity aerobic physical activity or 75 minutes of vigorous intensity aerobic activity every week.[30] Forty minutes of moderate to vigorous activity 3 to 4 days per week are recommended to improve blood pressure control and blood cholesterol levels. A minimum of 150 minutes per week of aerobic physical activity is recommended to address overweight and obesity, and 200 to 300 minutes per week of aerobic physical activity are recommended to help maintain long-term weight loss.[24]

MI is an effective tool for counseling patients regarding physical activity. A recent randomized controlled trial demonstrated MI as effective for long-term improvement in behavioral (walking for physical activity) and biomedical (cholesterol levels) CVD risk-associated outcomes.[31] Physical activity benefits are similar for patients of all ages and genders. Although women may derive even greater noncardiovascular benefit from physical activity (through mitigation of osteoporosis and depression), they are less likely to engage in regular physical activity.[27]

DIETARY INTAKE

There is controversy surrounding dietary patterns that specifically help to prevent CVD. Americans often struggle to adhere to heart-healthy diets (**Fig. 1**).[24] High intakes of fruits, vegetables, legumes, whole grains, low-fat dairy products, poultry, fish, nontropical vegetable oils, and nuts and limited consumption of sweets, sugar-sweetened beverages, salty or highly processed foods, and fatty red meats are recommended.[24] In general, patients are more likely to understand and follow advice focusing on foods to eat, or to avoid, rather than advice that is focused on individual nutrients (fats, carbohydrates, protein, sodium). Information about foods that are easily located while grocery shopping and easy to use for meal preparation facilitates counseling. **Table 3** compares the Mediterranean diet, the Dietary Approaches to Stop Hypertension (DASH) diet, and the AHA heart-healthy eating pattern.

Dietary Approaches to Stop Hypertension Diet

The DASH diet emphasizes fruits, vegetables, low-fat dairy products, whole grains, poultry, fish, and nuts. It promotes reduced intake of saturated fats, red meat, sweets,

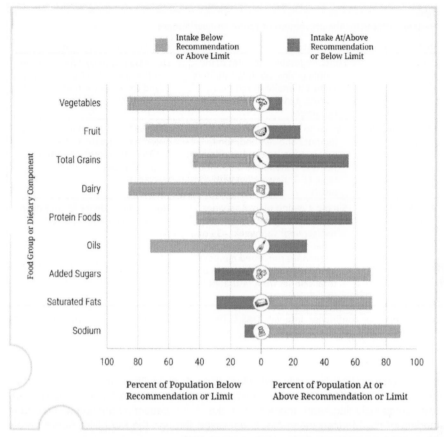

Fig. 1. Dietary intakes compared with recommendations. Percent of the US population 1 year of age and older who are lower than, at, or higher than each dietary goal or limit. Note that the *center (0) line* is the goal or limit. For most, those represented by the *orange* sections of the bars, shifting toward the *center line* improves their eating pattern. Data sources: What We Eat in America, National Health and Nutrition Examination Survey, 2007 to 2010, for average intakes by age-sex group. Healthy US-Style Food Patterns, which vary based on age, sex, and activity level, for recommended intakes and limits. From the 2015–2020 Dietary Guidelines for Americans and Report of the Dietary Guidelines Advisory Committee on the Dietary Guidelines of Americans 2015 to the Secretary of Agriculture and the Secretary of Health and Human Services. (*From* Van Horn L, Carson JAS, Appel LJ, et al. Recommended dietary pattern to achieve adherence to the AHA/ACC guidelines. Circulation 2016;134:e506; with permission.)

and sugar-sweetened beverages.[32] The DASH diet is a proven dietary approach to reduce blood pressure[32] and can also decrease the risk of coronary disease.[33] Adherence to the DASH diet is assessed with the Rate your Plate tool (http://www.dashdietoregon.org/Rate-Your-Plate).

Mediterranean Diet

The Mediterranean diet is similar to the DASH diet with an enhanced focus on legume consumption, moderate whole egg use, olive oil as the principal fat, and a moderate

Table 3
Dietary patterns for the prevention of cardiovascular disease

Dietary Pattern	Diet Content	CVD Prevention Outcomes
DASH	Fruits, vegetables, low-fat dairy, whole grains, poultry, fish, nuts. Reduced intake of red meat, sweets, and sugar-sweetened beverages	Decrease risk of coronary disease (RR = 0.79; 95% CI, 0.71–0.88) and stroke (RR = 0.81; 95% CI, 0.72–0.92)
Mediterranean diet	Similar to DASH with more legumes and seafood, some whole eggs, olive oil as primary fat, and a moderate amount of wine (1–2 glasses/day) with meals	29%–69% reduction in the risk of coronary disease and a 13%–53% reduction in the risk of stroke
AHA Healthy Heart	Simple 7 eating plan; 4 servings fruits and vegetables/day, nuts, two servings fish/week, <36 oz sugar-sweetened beverages/wk, <2 servings processed meats/wk, <1500 mg sodium/day, <7% of total calories from saturated fat/day	No specific evidence for this newly developed dietary pattern

Abbreviations: CI, confidence interval; DASH, Dietary Approaches to Stop Hypertension; RR, relative risk.
Data from Refs.[24,32–35]

alcohol consumption (typically red wine) (**Box 1**).[34] Multiple studies suggest that adherence to a Mediterranean-style diet is associated with a reduction in cardiovascular events including heart attack and stroke.[24,35] A patient's adherence and understanding of the Mediterranean diet is assessed through the Med Diet Score (http://oldwayspt.org/traditional-diets/mediterranean-diet).

Box 1
Characteristics of a Mediterranean dietary pattern

Fresh, minimally processed foods

Legumes

Fruits and vegetables

Whole grains

More seafood and poultry and minimal red meat

Nuts (walnuts, almonds, hazelnuts)

Two to four eggs per week

Moderate amount of dairy

Olive oil used for cooking

Fresh fruit for dessert

Moderate intake (1–2 glasses/day) of wine (red > white) with meals

Data from Refs.[24,34,35]

American Heart Association Heart-Healthy Eating Pattern

The AHA guidelines for healthy eating focus on foods to consume or avoid rather than on nutrient content. The Simple 7 guidelines recommend at least four servings of fruits and vegetables per day, four flat handfuls of nuts per week, and fish on at least 2 days per week.[9] These guidelines also recommend limiting sugar-sweetened beverages intake to less than 36 ounces per week, fewer than two servings of processed meats per week, less than 1500 mg of sodium per day, and less than 7% of total calories from saturated fat per day.[9] The AHA has also published a table that can be given to patients that contrasts foods to consume versus foods to avoid (**Table 4**).[24]

LIPID MANAGEMENT

The evidence to support lowering of low-density lipoprotein (LDL) cholesterol for secondary prevention of CVD is strong.[7,36] Historically, guidelines targeted treatment intensity based on specific LDL goals. Several, including AHA/ACC guidelines, the Veterans Affairs/Department of Defense guideline for the management of dyslipidemia, the United Kingdom National Institute for Health and Care Excellence guidance,

Table 4
Combining recommendations to help achieve a preferred heart-healthy dietary pattern

Foods to Encourage	Foods to Displace
Vegetables (fresh/frozen/canned without salt or rinsed; roasted/microwaved/stir-fried in unsaturated oil/steamed)	Vegetables with sauces/fried
Fruits (fresh/frozen/dried/canned without added sweetener, canned in juice)	Fruit pies, jams and jellies, fruit juice with added sugar
Whole grains and grains high in dietary fiber	Refined products (breads, white rice, cookies, granola bars, sugar-laden cereal, crackers, cakes) with added sugars and no or little fiber and/or solid fats
Low-fat and nonfat milk, dairy products, calcium-fortified nondairy milks	Full-fat dairy products
Poultry (skinless; grilled/baked/broiled)	Poultry with skin, fried poultry
Fish and seafood (grilled with unsaturated oils/baked/broiled)	Fish (battered and fried, buttered)
Legumes (beans, peas), sweet potatoes	French fries, white rice, white bread
Liquid vegetable oils (nontropical), soft margarines, stick margarines that have the same fatty acid profile as liquid vegetable oils	Butter, coconut, palm, and palm-kernel oils (tropical), traditional partially hydrogenated fat
Unsalted nuts and seeds; cut vegetables or fruit; baked, low-sodium chips; unsalted popcorn	Salted or candy-coated nuts and seeds, crackers, chips
Water and beverages without added sugars	Sugar-sweetened beverages, soda, presweetened teas, fruit drinks, sports drinks, energy drinks
Lean meat	Processed meat/sausage/hot dogs

From Van Horn L, Carson JAS, Appel LJ, et al. Recommended dietary pattern to achieve adherence to the AHA/ACC guidelines. Circulation 2016;134:e516; with permission.

and the American Diabetes Association (ADA) guidelines have recently shifted focus to emphasize global CVD risk reduction using foundational lifestyle change. Several others, including the Cochrane Collaboration and the US Preventive Services Task Force, have endorsed the treatment of hyperlipidemia in primary prevention to reduce the occurrence of CVD events.[5,37,38] In general, most guidelines (**Table 5**) currently recommend the use of statins as the primary pharmacologic intervention and match treatment intensity to the level of CVD risk.[7,8,39,40] They also demonstrate acceptable cost-effectiveness for the use of statins in primary prevention.[42]

For point-of-care use, the current ACC/AHA guideline, in particular, is accurate and efficient to help identify patients at increased risk for CVD.[43] The ACC/AHA determines global CVD risk and recommends lifestyle optimization focusing on tobacco avoidance, weight management, healthy eating, and at least 150 minutes of moderate aerobic activity each week.

Lipid-Lowering Therapy: Statins

Statins are the primary medication for the pharmacologic reduction of CVD risk because of their proven benefits at reducing LDL cholesterol and cardiovascular morbidity and mortality in primary and secondary prevention trials.[5,36,38] Statins are generally well tolerated with the most commonly reported side effect being muscle pain. Of note, in the large clinical trials of statins, muscle pain was reported slightly more commonly in those on placebo compared with statins.[44,45] Statin side effects,

Table 5 Comparison of four recent cholesterol reduction guidelines				
	ACC/AHA (2013)	**VA/DoD (2014)**	**NICE (2014)**	**ADA (2015)**
Risk calculator	Pooled cohort risk calculator	Any 10-y risk calculator	QRISK 2	No preference
Lifestyle changes	Foundational	Foundational	Foundational	Assumed
Lipid targets	No numerical LDL goal; treat to risk	No numerical LDL goal; treat to risk	No numerical LDL goal; treat to risk	No numerical LDL goal; treat to risk
Secondary prevention	High-dose statin to reduce LDL >50%	Moderate-dose statin	High-dose statin	High-dose statin to reduce LDL >50%
LDL ≥190 mg/dL	High-dose statin to reduce LDL >50%	Moderate-dose statin	High-dose statin	High-dose statin to reduce LDL >50%
Diabetes	Moderate to high dose based on overall CVD risk	Moderate-dose statin	Use statin for non-HDL-C reduction of ≥40%	Moderate to high dose based on overall CVD risk
Older adults	Not routinely indicated for age >75 y	Treat unless life expectancy <5 y	Treat as above <age 85; individualize >85 y	Same as above regardless of age
Monitoring	Initially at 12 wk; then every 3–12 mo	No routine monitoring	At 12 wk to assess reduction; then annually	Monitor as needed

Abbreviations: DoD, Department of Defense; NICE, National Institute for Health and Care Excellence; VA, Veterans Affairs.
Data from Refs.[7,8,39–41]

when they occur, are agent specific and not class specific.[44,45] The Food and Drug Administration no longer recommends the use of routine liver function monitoring in patients on statin therapy.[46]

Statins are recommended for prevention of CVD in patients with clinical CVD, those with an LDL-C greater than or equal to 190 mg/dL, patients aged 40 to 75 years with diabetes, and for patients with a 10-year CVD risk greater than or equal to 7.5%.[7] Individualized treatment with statins is recommended for patients with a 10-year risk between 5% and 7.5% and those with less than or equal to 5% 10-year risk with other significant cardiovascular risk (family history, elevated high-sensitivity C-reactive protein [hs-CRP] $\geq$2 mg/L, elevated coronary calcification score [CAC] $\geq$300 Agatson units, ankle brachial index [ABI] <0.9, or elevated lifetime risk of CVD) **(Fig. 2, Table 6)**.[7]

Nonstatin Medications

The addition of ezetimibe to a statin may also aid in secondary prevention.[47] Niacin and fibrates reduce triglycerides and LDL and raise HDL cholesterol, but have not been shown to reduce cardiovascular risk and are no longer recommended.[48] There is also no definitive evidence to support the use of fish oil supplements for the prevention of CVD.[48] The PCSK9 inhibitors, alirocumab and evolocumab, are the newest and highest potency class of medications for the reduction of LDL cholesterol. They are indicated for use when maximum dose statins do not lower LDL cholesterol sufficiently, or when a patient has a documented intolerance to statins. The addition of one of these medications to a statin can lower LDL an additional 50% to 60%.[49,50]

Patients on pharmacologic therapy should have lipid levels re-evaluated at 12 weeks with a focused medical history to assess compliance with medication and lifestyle changes. Annual follow-up is advised to ensure sufficient reduction in LDL cholesterol, assess medication compliance, and promote ongoing maintenance of lifestyle changes.[41]

HYPERTENSION MANAGEMENT

The risk of CVD begins at a blood pressure of 115/75 mm Hg and doubles with each incremental rise of 20/10 mm Hg.[51] The benefits of controlling blood for CVD prevention are well-established and founded on lifestyle management **(Box 2)**.[10,15,52,53]

The decision to start medical management depends on an individual's blood pressure level and cardiovascular risk. Patients with a systolic blood pressure (SBP) of 120 to 130 mm Hg or a diastolic blood pressure (DBP) of 80 to 89 mm Hg are considered prehypertensive and should be counseled on health-promoting lifestyle modifications to prevent CVD.[51] The Joint National Committee-8 Evidence-Based Guidelines for the Management of High blood pressure in adults provide nine key recommendations.[54] For the general population younger than 60 years of age, pharmacologic therapy should be initiated at a SBP greater than or equal to 140 mm Hg and/or DPB greater than or equal to 90 mm Hg and titrated to a goal DBP less than 90 mm Hg and less than 140 mm Hg. For patients older than the age of 60, pharmacologic therapy is recommended for an SBP greater than or equal to 150 mm Hg or DBP greater than or equal to 90 mm Hg. All patients older than 18 with chronic kidney disease and/or diabetes should start pharmacologic therapy at an SBP greater than or equal to 140 mm Hg and/or DPB greater than or equal to 90 mm Hg and treat to a goal DBP less than 90 mm Hg and less than 140 mm Hg. Combination treatment is needed to control blood pressure in most patients. A recent American College of Physician/American Academy of Family

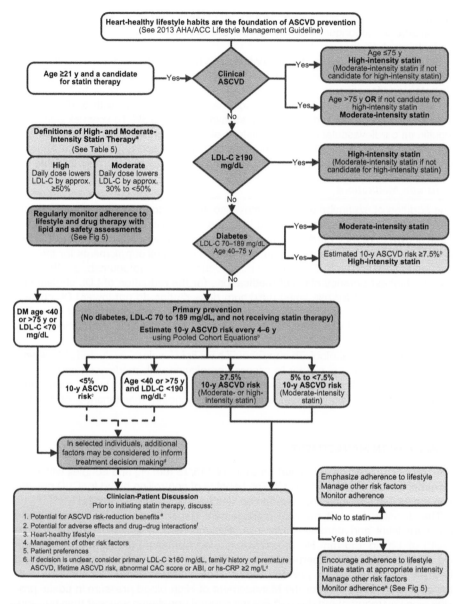

Fig. 2. Summary of statin initiation recommendations for the treatment of blood cholesterol to reduce ASCVD risk in adults. Assessment of the potential for benefit and risk from statin therapy for ASCVD prevention provides the framework for clinical decision making incorporating patient preferences. [a] Percent reduction in LDL-C can be used as an indication of response and adherence to therapy, but is not in itself a treatment goal. [b] The Pooled Cohort Equations can be used to estimate 10-year ASCVD risk in individuals with and without diabetes. The estimator within this application should be used to inform decision making in primary prevention patients not on a statin. [c] Consider moderate-intensity statin as more appropriate in low-risk individuals. [d] For those in whom a risk assessment is uncertain, consider such factors as primary LDL-C ≥160 mg/dL or other evidence of genetic hyperlipidemias; family history of premature ASCVD with

Table 6
Moderate- and high-intensity statin treatment

	High Intensity Reduce LDL >50%	Moderate Intensity Reduce LDL 30%–50%
Atorvastatin	40–80 mg/d	10–20 mg/d
Rosuvastatin	20–40 mg/d	5–10 mg/d
Simvastatin	Not safe (doses of 80 mg/d)	20–40 mg/d
Pravastatin	Not possible	40–80 mg/d
Lovastatin	Not possible	40 mg/d

Data from Stone NJ, Robinson JG, Lichtenstein AH, et al; American College of Cardiology/American Heart Association Task Force on Practice Guidelines. 2013 ACC/AHA guideline on the treatment of blood cholesterol to reduce atherosclerotic cardiovascular risk in adults: a report of the American College of Cardiology/American Heart Association Task Force on Practice Guidelines. Circulation 2014;129(25 Suppl 2):S1–45.

Physicians guideline recommends that lower SBP threshold (140 mm Hg) for initiating or intensifying pharmacologic therapy in adults aged 60 years or older with a history of stroke, transient ischemic attack, or at high cardiovascular risk.[55]

For the general population, benefits of treatment are based on absolute blood pressure reduction, rather than a specific drug type.[10,54] There are, however, several caveats. In black patients (including those with diabetes), initial antihypertensive treatment should include a thiazide-type diuretic or calcium channel blocker.[54] In patients with chronic kidney disease who are older than age 18, initial treatment should include an angiotensin-converting enzyme inhibitor or angiotensin receptor blocker.[54] The ADA further recommends that all patients with diabetes and hypertension should

---

onset <55 years of age in a first-degree male relative or <65 years of age in a first-degree female relative; hs-CRP ≥2 mg/L; CAC score ≥300 Agatston units or ≥75th percentile for age, sex, and ethnicity (for additional information, see http://www.mesa-nhlbi.org/CACReference.aspx); ABI <0.9; or lifetime risk of ASCVD. Additional factors that may aid in individual risk assessment may be identified in the future. [e] Potential ASCVD risk-reduction benefits. The absolute reduction in ASCVD events from moderate- or high-intensity statin therapy is approximated by multiplying the estimated 10-year ASCVD risk by the anticipated relative-risk reduction from the intensity of statin initiated (~30% for moderate-intensity statin or ~45% for high-intensity statin therapy). The net ASCVD risk-reduction benefit is estimated from the number of potential ASCVD events prevented with a statin, compared with the number of potential excess adverse effects. [f] Potential adverse effects. The excess risk of diabetes is the main consideration in ~0.1 excess cases per 100 individuals treated with a moderate-intensity statin for 1 year and ~0.3 excess cases per 100 individuals treated with a high-intensity statin for 1 year. In RCTs, statin-treated and placebo-treated participants experienced the same rate of muscle symptoms. The actual rate of statin-related muscle symptoms in the clinical population is unclear. Muscle symptoms attributed to statin therapy should be evaluated. ASCVD, atherosclerotic cardiovascular disease; LDL-C, low-density lipoprotein cholesterol; MI, myocardial infarction; RCT, randomized controlled trial. (*From* Stone NJ, Robinson JG, Lichtenstein AH, et al; American College of Cardiology/American Heart Association Task Force on Practice Guidelines. 2013 ACC/AHA guideline on the treatment of blood cholesterol to reduce atherosclerotic cardiovascular risk in adults: a report of the American College of Cardiology/American Heart Association Task Force on Practice Guidelines. Circulation 2014;129(25 Suppl 2):S9; with permission.)

Box 2
Recommendations for lifestyle management for blood pressure lowering

Consume a dietary pattern that emphasizes intake of vegetables, fruits, and whole grains; includes low-fat dairy products, poultry, fish, legumes, nontropical vegetable oils, and nuts; and limits intakes of sweets, sugar-sweetened beverages, and red meats
- Adapt this dietary pattern to appropriate calorie requirements, personal and cultural food preferences, and nutritional therapy for other medical conditions (including diabetes)
- Achieve this pattern following plans, such as the DASH dietary pattern, the US Department of Agriculture Food Pattern, or the AHA diet

Lower sodium intake

Consume no more than 2400 mg of sodium/d
- Further reductions of sodium intake to 1500 mg/d can result in even great reduction in blood pressure; and
- Even without achieving these goals, reducing sodium by at least 1000 g/d lowers blood pressure

Combine the DASH dietary pattern with lower sodium intake

Advise adults to engage in aerobic physical activity to lower blood pressure: three to four sessions per week, lasting on average 40 minutes per session, and involving moderate-to-vigorous intensity physical activity

Data from Eckel RH, Jakicic JM, Ard JD, et al. 2013 AHA/ACC guideline on lifestyle management to reduce cardiovascular risk: report of the American College of Cardiology/American Heart Association task force on practice guidelines. J Am Coll Cardiol 2014;63:2960–84.

---

be treated with either an angiotensin-converting enzyme inhibitor or angiotensin receptor blocker.[56]

There has been recent debate about whether or not patients with cardiovascular risk factors should receive intensive pharmacologic treatment to achieve a blood pressure less than 120/80 mm Hg.[57,58] The SPRINT trial suggests a more aggressive SBP target in select patients (eg, those aged 75 years or older with hypertension and no diabetes) with careful, frequent monitoring and follow-up.[59] The HOPE-3 trial, suggested a significant reduction in cardiovascular events in patients with uncomplicated, grade I hypertension with modest blood pressure lowering and simultaneous statin treatment. This less aggressive approach may be more readily incorporated into most clinical settings.[58,60]

GLUCOSE MANAGEMENT

Diabetes and prediabetes are independent risk factors for CVD.[56,61] Screening for abnormal blood glucose is recommended as a component of cardiovascular risk assessment in asymptomatic adults, aged 40 to 70 years who are either overweight or obese.[62] Earlier screening may be considered in patients with a family history of diabetes, a personal history of gestational diabetes or polycystic ovarian syndrome, and/or members of high-risk racial/ethnic groups (eg, African American, Latino, Native American, Asian American or Pacific Islander).[62] The ADA further recommends testing overweight or obese patients with a history of CVD, hypertension, HDL cholesterol less than 35 mg/dL, triglyceride level greater than 250 mg/dL, inactivity, or evidence of insulin resistance (eg, acanthosis nigricans).[63]

Lifestyle interventions are the cornerstones for managing prediabetes and the primary prevention of type 2 diabetes. Lifestyle modification is more effective than the use of medication to prevent progression to type 2 diabetes. There is an inverse association between activity levels and the risk of a cardiovascular event.[64] The Diabetes Prevention Program Study demonstrated that the onset of diabetes could be prevented or significantly delayed in high-risk patients who were able to achieve and maintain a minimum of 7% weight loss and 150 minutes of physical activity per week (eg, brisk walking 30 min/day, 5 day/wk).[65] Other cardiovascular risk factors, including decreased blood pressure, increased HDL cholesterol levels, and lower triglyceride levels, were reduced during 3-year follow-up.[66]

In addition to lifestyle changes, a variety of pharmacologic agents including metformin, α-glucosidase inhibitors, orlistat, glucagon-like peptide-1 receptor agonists, and thiazolidinediones have been shown to reduce the incidence of diabetes in patients with prediabetes.[67] The ADA recommends metformin to prevent diabetes in patients with prediabetes, particularly those who have a BMI greater than or equal to 35 kg/m^2, are younger than age 60, women with prior gestational diabetes mellitus, and/or patients with worsening prediabetes despite lifestyle intervention.[67] The key element to prevention seems to be specific changes in lifestyle because interventions focusing solely on weight loss have not consistently demonstrated reduced rates of cardiovascular events.[68]

In newly diagnosed patients with type 2 diabetes, more intense treatment may reduce long-term cardiovascular complications.[69] In contrast, intensive glycemic control trials involving patients with more advanced disease states have not demonstrated a consistent reduction in CVD outcomes and the risks of intensive control may outweigh the benefits. The ADA, therefore, recommends glycemic targets based on individualized patient goals.[69]

ASPIRIN

Recommendations regarding aspirin for CVD prevention are predicated on the patient's 10-year CVD risk balanced with the risk for bleeding complications. The ACC/AHA pooled cohort equation should be used to assess the 10-year risk for CVD.[70] The recommended dosage of aspirin is 81 mg per day **Table 7**.[70] Low-dose aspirin is recommended for CVD prevention in adults whose 10-year risk for a cardiovascular event exceeds 10%.[71]

Table 7 Usage of aspirin for cardiovascular disease prevention	
Category	Recommendation
Adults <50 y of age	No recommendation
Adults 50–59 y w/≥10%, 10-y risk for CVD, no increased bleeding risk, and life expectancy of 10 y	Administer 81 mg of daily aspirin
Adults 60–69 y w/≥10%, 10-y risk for CVD, no increased bleeding risk, and life expectancy of 10 y	Individualize treatment with 81 mg of daily aspirin based on life expectancy, patient desires, and comorbidity
Adults >70 y of age	No recommendation

Data from Bibbins-Domingo K, U.S. Preventive Services Task Force. Aspirin use for the primary prevention of cardiovascular disease and colorectal cancer: US Preventive Services Task Force recommendation statement. Ann Intern Med 2016;164(12): 836–45.

SUMMARY

CVD prevention requires an individualized and integrated approach to risk factor reduction. The AHA Simple 7 provides a framework to approach necessary changes. Even small incremental changes in lifestyle can have profound health benefits. A therapeutic partnership across time using targeted education, MI, and selected pharmacologic treatments can help significantly reduce CVD risk and burden of disease.

REFERENCES

1. Benjamin EJ, Blaha MJ, Chiuve SE, et al. Heart disease and stroke statistics – 2017 update: a report from the American Heart Association. Circulation 2017;135(10):e146–603.
2. Capewell S, Ford ES, Croft JB, et al. Cardiovascular risk factor trends and potential for reducing coronary heart disease mortality in the United States of America. Bull World Health Organ 2010;88(2):120–30.
3. Shay CM, Ning H, Allen NB, et al. Status of cardiovascular health in US adults; Prevalence estimates from the National Health and Nutrition Examination Surveys (NHANES). Circulation 2012;125:45–56.
4. Khanji MY, Bicalho VV, van Waardhuizen CN, et al. Cardiovascular risk assessment: a systematic review of guidelines. Ann Intern Med 2016;165(10):713–22.
5. US Preventive Services Task Force, Bibbins-Domingo K, Grossman DC, et al. Statin use for the primary prevention of cardiovascular disease in adults: US Preventive Services Task Force Recommendation Statement. JAMA 2016;316(19): 1997–2007.
6. Chou R, Dana T, Blazina I, et al. Screening for dyslipidemia in younger adults: a systematic review for the U.S. Preventive Services Task Force. Ann Intern Med 2016;165(8):560–4.
7. Stone NJ, Robinson JG, Lichtenstein AH, et al, American College of Cardiology/ American Heart Association Task Force on Practice Guidelines. 2013 ACC/AHA guideline on the treatment of blood cholesterol to reduce atherosclerotic cardiovascular risk in adults: a report of the American College of Cardiology/American Heart Association Task Force on Practice Guidelines. Circulation 2014;129(25 Suppl 2):S1–45.
8. National Institute for Health and Care Excellence (NICE). Guidelines for the reduction of cardiovascular disease risk. 2014: CG181. Available at: http://www.nice.org.uk/Guidance/CG181/Evidence. Accessed August 12, 2014.
9. Lloyd-Jones DM, Hong Y, Labarthe D, et al. Defining and setting national goals for cardiovascular health promotion and disease reduction: the American Heart Association's strategic Impact goal through 2020 and beyond. Circulation 2010;121:586–613.
10. Authors/Task Force Members, Piepoli MF, Hoes AW, et al. 2016 European guidelines on cardiovascular disease prevention in clinical practice: the sixth Joint Task Force of the European Society of Cardiology and other societies on cardiovascular disease prevention in clinical practice (constituted by representatives of 10 societies and by invited experts): developed with the special contribution of the European Association for Cardiovascular Prevention & Rehabilitation (EACPR). Eur J Prev Cardiol 2016;23(11):NP1–96.
11. National Institute for Health and Care Excellence (NICE). Guidelines for the reduction of cardiovascular disease risk. 2014: CG181. Available at: http://www.nice.org.uk/Guidance/CG181/Evidence. Accessed February 26, 2017.

12. WHO. Package of essential noncommunicable (PEN) disease interventions for primary healthcare in low-resource settings. Geneva (Switzerland): World Health Organization; 2010. Available at: http://apps.who.int/medicinedocs/documents/s19715en/s19715en.pdf. Accessed February 26, 2017.

13. Ford ES, Greenlund KJ, Hong Y. Ideal cardiovascular health and mortality from all causes and disease of the circulatory system among adults in the United States. Circulation 2012;125:987–95.

14. Younus A, Aneni EC, Spatz ES, et al. A systematic review of the prevalence and outcomes of ideal cardiovascular health in US and non-US populations. Mayo Clin Proc 2016;91:649–70.

15. Ogunmoroti O, Allen NB, Cushman M, et al. Association between Life's Simple 7 and noncardiovascular disease: the multi-ethnic study of atherosclerosis. J Am Heart Assoc 2016;5:e003954.

16. Larzelere MM, Williams DE. Promoting smoking cessation. Am Fam Physician 2012;85(6):591–8.

17. Fiore MC, Jaén CR, Baker TB, et al. Treating tobacco use and dependence: 2008 update. Clinical practice guideline. Rockville (MD): U.S. Department of Health and Human Services. Public Health Service; 2008. Available at: https://www.ncbi.nlm.nih.gov/books/NBK63952/. Accessed April 7, 2017.

18. Lindson-Hawley N, Thompson TP, Begh R. Motivational interviewing for smoking cessation. Cochrane Database Syst Rev 2015;(3):CD006936.

19. Rothemich SF, Woolf SH, Johnson RE, et al. Effect on cessation counseling of documenting smoking status as a routine vital sign: an ACORN study. Ann Fam Med 2008;6(1):60–8.

20. Hughes JR, Stead LF, Hartmann-Boyce J, et al. Antidepressants for smoking cessation. Cochrane Database Syst Rev 2014;((1):CD000031.

21. Gonzales D, Rennard SI, Nides M, et al. Varenicline, an alpha4beta2 nicotinic acetylcholine receptor partial agonist, vs sustained-release bupropion and placebo for smoking cessation: a randomized controlled trial. JAMA 2006;296(1):47–55.

22. US Food and Drug Administration. FDA Drug Safety Communication: Chantix (varenicline) drug label now contains updated efficacy and safety information. 2011. Available at: https://www.fda.gov/Drugs/DrugSafety/ucm264436.htm. Accessed April 5, 2017.

23. Stead LF, Hartmann-Boyce J, Perera R, et al. Telephone counselling for smoking cessation. Cochrane Database Syst Rev 2013;(8):CD002850.

24. Van Horn L, Carson JA, Appel LJ, et al. Recommended dietary pattern to achieve adherence to the American Heart Association/American College of Cardiology (AHA/ACC) Guidelines: a scientific statement from the American Heart Association. Circulation 2016;134(22):e505–29.

25. Office of Disease Prevention and Health Promotion. Report of the dietary guidelines advisory committee on the dietary guidelines of Americans 2015 to the Secretary of Agriculture and the Secretary of Health and Human Services. Available at: https://health.gov/dietaryguidelines/2015-scientific-report/. Accessed December 27, 2016.

26. Zogbhi WA, Holmes DR. Improving cardiovascular health. JAMA 2013;309:1117–9.

27. Hivert MF, Arena R, Forman DE, et al. Medical training to achieve competency in lifestyle counseling: an essential foundation for prevention and treatment of cardiovascular diseases and other chronic medical conditions: a scientific statement from the American Heart Association. Circulation 2016;134(15):e308–27.

28. Burke LE, Wang J, Sevick MA. Self-monitoring in weight loss: a systematic review of the literature. J Am Diet Assoc 2011;111(1):92–102.
29. Donaldson JM, Normand MP. Using goal setting, self-monitoring, and feedback to increase calorie expenditure in obese adults. Behav Intervent 2009;24:73–83.
30. Lanier JB, Bury DC, Richardson SW. Diet and physical activity for cardiovascular disease prevention. Am Fam Physician 2016;93(11):919–24.
31. Hardcastle SJ, Taylor AH, Bailey MP, et al. Effectiveness of a motivational interviewing intervention on weight loss, physical activity and cardiovascular disease risk factors: a randomized controlled trial with a 12-month post-intervention follow-up. Int J Behav Nutr Phys Act 2013;10:40.
32. Svetkey LP, Simons-Morton D, Vollmer WM, et al. Effects of dietary patterns on blood pressure: subgroup analysis of the dietary approaches to stop hypertension (DASH) randomized clinical trial. Arch Intern Med 1999;159:285–93.
33. Salehi-Abargouei A, Maghsoudi Z, Shirani F, et al. Effects of dietary approaches to stop hypertension (DASH)-style diet on fatal or nonfatal cardiovascular diseases incidence – a systematic review and meta-analysis on observational prospective studies. Nutrition 2013;29(4):611–8.
34. Walker C, Reamy BV. Diets for cardiovascular disease prevention: what is the evidence? Am Fam Physician 2009;79(7):571–8.
35. Estruch R, Ros E, Salas-Salvado J, et al. Primary prevention of cardiovascular disease with a Mediterranean diet. N Engl J Med 2013;368:1279–90.
36. Skinner JS, Cooper A. Secondary prevention of ischaemic cardiac events. Clin Evid 2009;09:206.
37. Mihaylova B, Emberson J, Blackwell L, et al. Cholesterol Treatment Trialists (CTT) Collaborators. The effects of lowering LDL cholesterol with statin therapy in people at low risk of vascular disease: meta-analysis of individual data form 27 randomized trials. Lancet 2012;380(9841):581–90.
38. Taylor F, Huffman MD, Macedo A, et al. Statins for the primary prevention of cardiovascular disease. Cochrane Database Syst Rev 2013;(1):CD004816.
39. Downs JR, O'Malley PG. Management of dyslipidemia for cardiovascular disease risk reduction: synopsis of the 2014 US Department of Veteran's Affairs and US Department of Defense clinical practice guidelines. Ann Intern Med 2015;163: 291–7.
40. American Diabetes Association. Cardiovascular disease and risk management. Diabetes Care 2015;38(Suppl 1):S49–57.
41. Ganda OP. Deciphering cholesterol treatment guidelines: a clinician's perspective. JAMA 2015;313(10):1009–10.
42. Pandya A, Sy S, Cho S, et al. Cost-effectiveness of 10-year risk thresholds for initiation of statin therapy for primary prevention of cardiovascular disease. JAMA 2015;314(2):142–50.
43. Pursnani A, Massaro JM, D'Agostino RB, et al. Guideline based statin eligibility, coronary artery calcification, and cardiovascular events. JAMA 2015;314(2): 134–41.
44. Guyton JR, Bays HE, Grundy SM, et al. An assessment by the statin intolerance panel: 2014 update. J Clin Lipidol 2014;8:S72–81.
45. Ganga HV, Slim HB, Thompson PD. A systematic review of statin induced muscle problems in clinical trials. Am Heart J 2014;168(1):6–15.
46. FDA Drug Safety Communication: important safety label changes to cholesterol-lowering statin drugs. 2012. Available at: http://www.fda.gov/Drugs/DrugSafety/ucm293101.htm. Accessed December 16, 2012.

47. Cannon CP, Blazing MA, Giugliano RP, et al. Ezetimibe added to statin therapy after acute coronary syndromes. N Engl J Med 2015;372(25):2387–97.
48. Lipid lowering drugs. Med Lett Drugs Ther 2016;58(1506):133–40.
49. Robinson JG, Farnier M, Krempf M, et al. Efficacy and safety of alirocumab in reducing lipids and cardiovascular events. N Engl J Med 2015;372(16):1489–99.
50. Sabatine MS, Giugliano RP, Wiviott SD, et al. Efficacy and safety of evolocumab in reducing lipids and cardiovascular events. N Engl J Med 2015;372(16):1500–9.
51. Chobanian AV, Bakris GL, Black HR, et al, National Heart, Lung and Blood Institute Joint National Committee on Prevention, Detection, Evaluation and Treatment of High Blood Pressure; National High blood Pressure Education Program Coordinating Committee. The seventh report of the Joint National Committee on prevention, detection, evaluation, and treatment of high blood pressure: the JNC 7 report. JAMA 2003;289:2560–72.
52. Ettehad D, Emdin C, Kiran A, et al. Blood pressure lowering for prevention of cardiovascular disease and death: a systematic review and meta-analysis. Lancet 2016;387:957–67.
53. Eckel RH, Jakicic JM, Ard JD, et al. 2013 AHA/ACC guideline on lifestyle management to reduce cardiovascular risk: a report of the American College of Cardiology/American Heart Association task force on practice guidelines. J Am Coll Cardiol 2014;63:2960–84.
54. James PA, Oparil S, Carter B, et al. 2014 evidence-based guidelines for the management of high blood pressure in adults: report from the panel members appointed to the eight joint national committee. JAMA 2014;311:507–20.
55. Qaseem A, Wilt TJ, Rich R, et al. Pharmacologic treatment of hypertension in adults aged 60 years or older to higher versus lower blood pressure targets: a clinical practice guideline from the American College of Physicians and the American Academy of Family Physicians. Ann Intern Med 2017;166:430–7.
56. American Diabetes Association. Cardiovascular disease and risk management. Diabetes Care 2017;40(Suppl 1):S75–87.
57. Oparil S, Lewis CE. Should patients with cardiovascular risk factors receive intensive treatment of hypertension to < 120/80 mm Hg target? A protagonists view from the SPRINT (systolic blood pressure intervention trial). Circulation 2016;134:1308–10.
58. Lonn EM, Yusuf S. Should patients with cardiovascular risk factors receive intensive treatment of hypertension to < 120/80 mm Hg target? An antagonist view from the HOPE-3 trial (Heart Outcomes Evaluation-3). Circulation 2016;134:1311–3.
59. Williamson JD, Supiano MA, Applegate WB, et al. Intensive vs standard blood pressure control and cardiovascular disease outcomes in adults aged ≥ 75 years: a randomized controlled trial. JAMA 2016;315:2673–82.
60. Lonn EM, Bosch J, Lopez-Jaramillo P, et al. Blood-pressure lowering in intermediate-risk persons without cardiovascular disease. N Engl J Med 2016;274:2009–20.
61. Huang Y, Xiaoyan C, Weiyi M, et al. Association between prediabetes and risk of cardiovascular disease and all-cause mortality: systematic review and meta-analysis. BMJ 2016;355:i5953.
62. Siu AL, US Preventive Services Task Force. Screening for abnormal blood glucose and type 2 diabetes mellitus: U.S. Preventive Services Task Force recommendation statement. Ann Intern Med 2015;163:861–8.
63. American Diabetes Association. Classification and diagnosis of diabetes. Diabetes Care 2017;40(Suppl 1):S11–24.

64. Yates T, Haffner SM, Schulte PJ, et al. Association between change in daily ambulatory activity and cardiovascular events in people with impaired glucose tolerance (NAVIGATOR trial): a cohort analysis. Lancet 2014;383:1059–66.

65. Findström J, Ilanne-Parikka P, Peltonen M, et al, Finnish Diabetes Prevention Study Group. Sustained reduction in the incidence of type 2 diabetes by lifestyle intervention: follow-up of the Finnish Diabetes Prevention Study. Lancet 2006;368: 1673–9.

66. The Diabetes Prevention Program Research Group. Impact of intensive lifestyle and metformin therapy on cardiovascular risk factors in the Diabetes Prevention Program. Diabetes Care 2005;28:888–94.

67. American Diabetes Association. Prevention or delay of type 2 diabetes. Diabetes Care 2017;40(Suppl 1):S44–7.

68. Look AHEAD Research Group. Cardiovascular effects of intensive lifestyle intervention in type 2 diabetes. N Engl J Med 2013;369:145–54.

69. American Diabetes Association. Glycemic targets. Diabetes Care 2017;40(Suppl 1):S48–56.

70. Bibbins-Domingo K, U.S. Preventive Services Task Force. Aspirin use for the primary prevention of cardiovascular disease and colorectal cancer: US Preventive Services Task Force recommendation statement. Ann Intern Med 2016;164(12): 836–45.

71. Goldstein LB, Bushnell CD, Adams RJ, et al. Guidelines for the primary prevention of stroke; a guideline for healthcare professionals from the American Heart Association/American Stroke Association. Stroke 2011;42:517–84.

Coronary Artery Disease
Diagnosis and Management

Stephen D. Cagle Jr, MD*, Noah Cooperstein, MD

KEYWORDS

- Coronary artery • Cardiovascular • Risk reduction • Prevention

KEY POINTS

- Primary and secondary prevention of cardiovascular events are central to the management of coronary artery disease (CAD).
- Many patients are asymptomatic. Prevention and treatment strategies are based on atherosclerotic cardiovascular disease (ASCVD) risk.
- Patients with stable angina should undergo a systematic evaluation, and those with acute chest pain or unstable angina (acute coronary syndromes) should be evaluated and managed in an emergency setting.
- Lifestyle modification is an integral part of risk reduction in patients with elevated ASCVD risk or known CAD.
- Statin therapy is a first line of pharmacotherapy for management of CAD.

INTRODUCTION

Coronary artery disease (CAD) is common. There are an estimated 660,000 to 750,000 cardiovascular events yearly in the United States. Approximately two-thirds of events are first-time events. Some type of cardiovascular event (acute coronary syndrome) occurs approximately every 43 seconds in the United States.[1,2] Risk stratification, assessment of patients with stable angina, and management of primary and secondary prevention of cardiovascular events are key components in caring for patients at risk of CAD and cardiovascular events (myocardial infarction [MI]/ischemia, angina, or stroke).

DEFINITION
Coronary Artery Disease

CAD is characterized by atherosclerosis in the epicardial coronary arteries. Atherosclerotic plaques narrow the coronary artery lumen, impairing the antegrade myocardial blood flow.[3]

Disclosure Statement: The authors have nothing to disclose.
Saint Louis University Family Medicine Residency - O' Fallon, 1 St. Elizabeth's Drive, Suite 400, O'Fallon, IL 62269, USA
* Corresponding author.
E-mail address: scaglejr@gmail.com

Prim Care Clin Office Pract 45 (2018) 45–61
https://doi.org/10.1016/j.pop.2017.10.001
0095-4543/18/Published by Elsevier Inc.

Coronary Heart Disease

Patients who have had MI, percutaneous coronary intervention (PCI), or coronary artery bypass graft have coronary heart disease (CHD).[4,5]

SYMPTOM CRITERIA

Many patients with CAD are asymptomatic when they present to the office. In this setting, screening is based on current guideline recommendations from the US Preventive Services Task Force (USPSTF), American College of Cardiology/American Heart Association (ACC/AHA), or American Association of Clinical Endocrinologists (AACE).[1,6,7] Patients are stratified and treated based on atherosclerotic cardiovascular disease (ASCVD) risk using a pooled cohort analysis tool, of which several are available.[1,6,7] Patients with CAD can also present with more familiar descriptions of chest pain, such as a squeezing or pressure sensation that occurs with exertion and is relieved with rest. These findings are consistent with CAD and require further workup and management.[1,3,6,7]

CLINICAL FINDINGS
Patient History

In patients without known CAD, a detailed history helps calculate the risk of having a cardiovascular event at some point in the future. The medical history also identifies relevant comorbidities and helps to rule out other causes in patients presenting with chest pain. The medical history should capture details of patient diet, physical activity, family history of heart disease, and a relevant social history, including occupation, and tobacco and alcohol use Strength of recommendation (SOR A). The patient interview can be guided in part by the 9 modifiable risk factors identified by the 2004 INTERHEART study (**Box 1**).[8] Discussion of social history should address not only smoking but also the use of recreational stimulants such as cocaine and methamphetamine (SOR A). Stimulants cause acute chest pain via coronary artery vasoconstriction and demand ischemia, and chronic

---

Box 1
INTERHEART Study: 9 potentially modifiable risk factors

- Smoking
- Hypertension
- Diabetes
- Abdominal obesity
- Stress and depression
- Daily consumption of fruits and vegetables
- Regular alcohol consumption
- Regular physical activity
- Dyslipidemia

Identified in case control study of nearly 30,000 participants in 52 countries.
Data from Yusuf S, Hawken S, Ôunpuu S, et al. Effect of potentially modifiable risk factors associated with myocardial infarction in 52 countries (the INTERHEART study): case-control study. Lancet 2004;364(9438):937–52.

---

cocaine use has been implicated in premature development of CAD.[9] Taking the history should also include looking for symptoms of depression and an inquiry about each patient's social support network. Recent evidence suggests that social isolation is an independent and significant risk factor for heart disease and stroke.[10] The patient interview also provides the opportunity to engage in shared decisions about future testing and treatment, including risks, benefits, and costs.[11]

Physical Examination

The broad differential diagnosis for chest pain warrants a systematic approach. In addition to ischemic cardiovascular chest pain, the differential should include nonischemic cardiovascular, pulmonary, gastrointestinal, musculoskeletal, and psychiatric causes of chest pain (**Table 1**).[12–14] These categories can guide history taking, physical examination, laboratory testing, and radiographic imaging.

The physical examination of patients with CAD is often unremarkable. The examination should include accurate measurement of blood pressure and calculation of body mass index, 2 fundamental measures of cardiovascular health (SOR A). Auscultation of heart and lungs and evaluation of skin and extremities are also important and can help identify comorbid conditions (**Table 2**). Other clues from the examination can aid in identifying comorbid conditions and other nonischemic causes of chest pain.[12] In those patients reporting recent chest pain, the physical examination can additionally help identify nonischemic cardiovascular causes of chest pain and noncardiovascular causes of chest discomfort (**Table 3**).

Screening: Cardiovascular Disease Risk Prediction Models

Relatively few American adults adhere to a healthy lifestyle. Lack of healthy lifestyle significantly increases the risk for cardiovascular disease at the population level. In a recent study of nearly 5000 US adults, fewer than 3 in 100 adults met 4 basic wellness criteria: adequate physical activity, consuming a healthy diet, no tobacco use, and falling within recommended body fat percentages.[15] Atherosclerotic CAD appears to start in childhood, with intimal coronary artery lesions found on autopsy in nearly half of apparently healthy 15- to 19-year-old subjects.[16] It is recommended, therefore, that modifiable risk factors for cardiovascular disease (see **Box 1**) be assessed every 4 to 6 years beginning at age 20 (SOR A).[17]

In addition to routine office-based screening for common risk factors, multiple clinical predictive models (CPMs) are available to help assess cardiovascular risk and guide primary prevention (**Table 4**).[18] The appropriate application of well-validated CPMs has the potential to improve individual outcomes and optimize resource utilization.[19] CPMs also allow patients the opportunity to actively participate in their disease management by helping them to better understand the risks and benefits of various treatment recommendations and strategies.[17]

One of the drawbacks of CPM is the controversy about fixed-term versus lifetime risk. Most CPMs offer a 10-year risk estimation. This 10-year risk, particularly in younger patients, is often much lower than lifetime risk. This may give patients a false sense of security regarding their overall cardiovascular risk.[20] Furthermore, external CPM validation is limited, and few have been tested in head-to-head comparisons against competing models.[18] In addition, several of the CPMs, including the AHA/ACC pooled cohort ASCVD risk calculator, have been shown to overestimate risk.[21] Although the potential clinical impact of these models remains poorly understood,[18,22] CMPs currently offer the most systematic approach to risk estimation and should therefore be used to guide the cardiovascular risk stratification (SOR A).

Table 1
Alternative diagnoses to angina for patients with chest pain

Ischemic Non-Atherosclerotic Artery Disease	Nonischemic Cardiovascular	Pulmonary	Gastrointestinal	Chest Wall	Psychiatric
Cocaine induced Vasospasm Prinzmetal angina	Aortic dissection Pericarditis Aortic stenosis	Pulmonary embolus Pneumothorax Pneumonia Pleuritis	Esophageal Esophagitis Spasm Reflux Biliary Colic Cholecystitis Choledocholithiasis Cholangitis Peptic ulcer Pancreatitis	Costochondritis Fibrositis Rib fracture Sternoclavicular arthritis Herpes zoster (before the rash)	Anxiety disorders Hyperventilation Panic disorder Primary anxiety Affective disorders (eg, depression) Somatoform disorders Thought disorders (eg, fixed delusions)

Data from Refs.[12–14]

Table 2	
Physical examination: finding of comorbid conditions	
Carotid bruits, decreased pedal pulses	Peripheral artery disease
Acanthosis nigricans	Insulin resistance
Pedal edema, pulmonary rales, JVD	Congestive heart failure
S4 heart sound	Left ventricular dysfunction, ventricular hypertrophy

Abbreviation: JVD, jugular venous distention.
  Data from Menees DS, Bates ER. Evaluation of patients with suspected coronary artery disease. Coron Artery Dis 2010;21(7):386–90.

Risk Estimation: Beyond Clinical Predictive Models

Thirty-year and lifetime risk
Most of the widely used CPMs calculate the 10-year absolute risk for a cardiovascular event. Thirty-year and lifetime cardiovascular risk are based on age, sex, total high-density lipoprotein cholesterol (HDL-C), blood pressure, the use of antihypertensive medications, the presence of diabetes, and tobacco use.[23] Based on data from the Framingham Heart Study, a 30-year ASVCD risk calculator is available online (https://www.framinghamheartstudy.org/risk-functions/cardiovascular-disease/30-year-risk.php#). Although less useful for guiding pharmacotherapy, the estimation of lifetime risk helps promote lifestyle modification in younger patients who have a substantial lifetime risk of CAD, but low 10-year risk.[17]

Electrocardiography
The USPSTF currently recommends against screening low-risk, asymptomatic adults for the prediction of cardiovascular events with either resting or exercise electrocardiography (ECG). The USPSTF also states that there is insufficient evidence to recommend resting or exercise ECG for screening of intermediate- and high-risk adults.[24]

Diabetes—risk predictor or risk equivalent?
There is active debate as to role diabetes mellitus (DM) in predicting CHD.[4] The Executive Summary of the Third Report of the National Cholesterol Education Program

Table 3	
Physical examination: findings of nonischemic cardiovascular pain and noncardiovascular pain	
Tachycardia, hypoxia, dyspnea	Pulmonary embolism
Irregular peripheral pulses	Supraventricular arrhythmia
Systolic murmur	Aortic stenosis Mitral valve regurgitation Hypertrophic obstructive cardiomyopathy
Friction rub, pain relieved by leaning forward	Pericarditis
Reproducible chest wall pain, especially along the costochondral margin	Costochondritis, other musculoskeletal cause
Pulmonary rhonchi, dullness to percussion, egophony, tactile fremitus	Pneumonia
Abdominal tenderness	Peptic ulcer disease, biliary colic, chronic pancreatitis

Data from Menees DS, Bates ER. Evaluation of patients with suspected coronary artery disease. Coron Artery Dis 2010;21(7):386–90.

Table 4
Clinical predictive models for atherosclerotic coronary artery disease

Name	End Points	Notes
2008, Framingham General CVD risk score (Agostino 2008)[67]	• Death from CHD • Nonfatal MI • Angina • CVA (fatal or nonfatal, ischemic, or hemorrhagic) • TIA • Claudication • Heart failure	This is an update of both the original 1998 and subsequent 2002 models
2007, Reynolds CVD Risk Score (Ridker 2007)[68]	• Cardiovascular death • Nonfatal MI • Nonfatal CVA • Coronary revascularization	Separate scoring for men and women. Uses high sensitivity CRP
2013, ACC/AHA Pooled Cohort ASCVD Risk Calculator (Goff 2014)[69]	• Death from CHD • Nonfatal MI • Angina • CVA (fatal or nonfatal, ischemic, or hemorrhagic) • TIA • Claudication • Heart failure	Recent evidence suggests significant overestimation of risk (Rana 2016)[21]
2015, MESA Risk Score (Budoff 2009)[70]	• Death from CHD • Nonfatal MI • Resuscitated cardiac arrest coronary revascularization	Designed to account for ethnic diversity beyond that seen in the original Framingham study population. Calculation also has option to include CAC scores

(NCEP) included DM as a CHD risk equivalent.[5] Other well-designed, large-scale studies disagree.[21,25] Recent guidelines list DM as a risk predictor rather than an equivalent.[17] In either case, DM elevates the absolute risk for cardiovascular disease (CVD) and should be screened for in all patients at risk for CHD (SOR A).[26]

Urine microalbumin

In asymptomatic patients without hypertension or diabetes, microalbuminuria (MA) is associated with increased risk of developing CHD. This is true even when low-grade MA is present at levels below the standard threshold of urine albumin to creatine ratio of 30 μg/mg.[27] In hypertensive patients, MA predicts not only cardiovascular risk but also a reduction of microalbumin through treatment with angiotensin converting enzyme (ACE) inhibitors reduces cardiovascular risk.[28] In diabetic patients, MA increases the risk of developing CHD above the baseline risk associated with diabetes alone.[29] Although MA has not been integrated into any widely used CPMs, clinicians should consider including MA as part of CVD risk assessment, especially in patients with hypertension or diabetes (SOR B).[26]

Advanced lipid profiling

The association between traditional lipid measures and the risk for CVD is covered elsewhere. In addition, recent research has focused on apolipoprotein markers for CVD. Apolipoproteins are amphipathic proteins that allow for the transport of insoluble lipids in blood plasma. Apolipoprotein A1 and apolipoprotein B (apoB) are associated with high density lipoproteins and low-density lipoproteins (LDL), respectively.[30] Although there is some evidence to support the use of apoB for risk stratification, meta-analyses on the subject are in conflict and the improvement in risk prediction appears nominal.[31] Hypertriglyceridemia with elevated abpoB is closely associated with diabetes and metabolic syndrome, but these overt conditions are themselves significant risk factors, if not risk equivalents, making the addition of apoB of little clinical value.[31-33]

C-reactive protein levels
Elevation of C-reactive protein (CRP) is associated with fatal and nonfatal CAD events and nonfatal peripheral artery disease events. Rather than using CRP as an independent CVD risk marker, it is more reliably applied as part of a more global CPM.[34] The Reynolds CVD Risk Score is one example of a model that incorporates CRP levels with other risk factors as part of a multivariate prediction.[35]

Coronary artery calcium scores
Coronary artery calcium (CAC) scores are obtained by chest computed tomography. Like CRP, they are also of greatest use when applied in the context of a CPM. The Multi-Ethnic Study of Atherosclerosis (MESA) Risk Score is one example.[36] CAC scores have a strong negative predictive value, helping to identify patients who do likely not benefit from lifelong preventive pharmacotherapy.[37]

B-type natriuretic peptide
Plasma concentrations of B-type natriuretic peptide (BNP) correlate strongly with cardiovascular risk. The predictive utility of BNP, however, remains unclear, and the most recent ACC/AHA guidelines recommend against BNP as a screening tool for CAD risk.[38]

Genetic testing
Many patients are genetically predisposed to CHD.[26] Numerous genome-wide variants and single nucleotide polymorphisms confer increased risk for CAD. To date, however, there is no preferred genetic test available to predict CVD risk in the general population. The most recent ACC/AHA guidelines recommend against genomic testing as a screen tool for CVD risk.[39,40]

Other biomarkers of cardiovascular risk
Eighteen other biomarkers in the broad categories of inflammation, hemostasis, hemodynamic stress, and ischemia have recently been identified as cardiovascular risk predictors.[41] Although promising, these biomarkers are currently of limited or unclear utility for routine use in predicting cardiovascular risk.

Coronary Heart Disease Risk Equivalents

A "risk equivalent" suggests that the likelihood for a major cardiovascular event is similar to either that of a previous MI or a 20% 10-year risk.[5] **Table 5** lists established CHD risk equivalents. As an example, patients who have suffered either a transient ischemic attack (TIA) or an ischemic cerebral vascular accident (CVA) have a roughly 2% annual risk of developing CHD. Over a 10-year period, this confers a 20% risk, making TIA or ischemic CVA a CHD risk equivalent.[42,43] Recent evidence has strongly suggested that chronic kidney disease (CKD) should be included as a CHD risk equivalent as well.[44,45] Patients with established CHD or a CHD risk equivalent do not require risk-factor screening. Instead, these individuals should be managed using secondary prevention guidelines.

Table 5
Coronary heart disease risk equivalents

Other clinical manifestations of atherosclerotic disease	These include peripheral artery disease, abdominal aortic aneurysm, symptomatic carotid artery disease, and intermittent claudication (NCEP 2001)
Multiple risk factors sufficient to confer a 10-y risk for developing CHD > 20%	For patients who report multiple risk factors but do not have a history of CHD or other manifestation of atherosclerotic disease, the application of a CPM is of use to determine risk (NCEP 2001)
TIA or ischemic CVA	Confers a 2% annual risk, which corresponds to a 20% 10-y risk (Amaremco et al,[71] 2008, Touze et al,[72] 2005)
CKD	10-y risk of cardiovascular events increases as kidney function declines (Tonelli et al,[45] 2012, Briasoulis & Bakris,[44] 2013)
DM	Although patients with DM are at higher risk for developing CHD, DM itself does not increase risk substantially enough to be considered a risk equivalent (Bulugahapitiya et al,[25] 2009, Rana et al,[73] 2016)

Diagnostic Testing

In contrast to routine screening, patients with recent or active chest pain should be evaluated using appropriate diagnostic testing. In these patients, a resting ECG should be obtained to establish baseline electrophysiology, identify left ventricular hypertrophy, old MI, acute ischemic changes, and any evidence of conduction abnormalities (SOR A).[12] In addition, clinical prediction rules can help determine the likelihood of obstructive CAD.[46]

Management

Management goals and treatment recommendations vary by professional societies. The USPSTF, ACC/AHA, and AACE use ASCVD risk calculators to determine when and how to initiate treatment.[1,7,17] Treatment targets and goals are presented in **Table 6**. The USPSTF offers recommendations for primary prevention only, whereas the AACE and the ACC/AHA have differing secondary prevention goals (**Table 7**). Implementation of guidelines helps identify individuals who need treatment.[47,48]

Pharmacologic Strategies

There are multiple classes of medications used to manage CAD and prevent future cardiovascular events (**Table 8**). Statin therapy is recommended as the first-line therapy for primary and secondary prevention of CVD by the USPSTF, ACC/AHA, and the AACE (see **Table 6**).[1,7,49] Specific recommendations vary by organization (**Table 9**). The approach to medication management should be individualized based on patient history and associated risk factors (SOR A).

Statins

HMG Co-A reductase inhibitors (statins) are categorized based on expected reduction in LDL. High-intensity statin therapy results in a greater than 50% reduction, moderate intensity 30% to 50% reduction, and low intensity a less than 30% reduction in serum LDL values.[17] Statin therapy is recommended for patients at high risk for CVD because they have been shown to benefit most from this treatment (SOR A). Patients in lower-risk categories benefit less from statin therapy, and routine may be harmful in low-risk elderly patients (SOR A). When determining the best management approach for low-risk patients, an individualized approach using shared decision making is most appropriate (SOR A). In addition, attention to secondary prevention has the most significant

Table 6		
Statin initiation based on guidelines		
Guideline	**Initiation**	**Qualifiers**
USPSTF	>10%	Aged 40–75 with 1 or more of following: 1. Dyslipidemia 2. Diabetes 3. Hypertension 4. Smoking
ACC/AHA	Any of the following: ≥7.5% ASCVD risk LDL-C >190 mg/dL DM	Aged 40–75
AACE	Low risk Moderate risk High risk	0 risk factors > LDL-C 130 mg/dL ≤2 risk factors and 10-y ASCVD risk of <10% ≥2 risk factors and 10-y ASCVD risk of 10%–20% Diabetes of CKD stage 3 or greater
	Very high risk	ASCVD 10-y risk >20% Diabetes, PVD, or CKD stage 3 or greater with 1 or more risk factors Familial hypercholesterolemia

Data from Refs.[1,7,45]

clinical benefit with dedicated statin use. Patients having known CHD or CHD risk equivalents benefit the most from aggressive statin therapy (SOR A).

Fibrates

Fibrates are often used as second-line agents for the management of ASCVD risk reduction. Their use is recommended by ACC/AHA and AACE if the patient's overall goal of risk reduction is not met.[1,49] A *Cochrane Review* found a less than 1% Absolute Risk Reduction for primary prevention of cardiovascular events and no effect on mortality.[50] A separate *Cochrane Review* for fibrates in secondary prevention that included 13 trials and 16,112 patients showed a decrease in nonfatal events, but no reduction in mortality.[51] Fibrates do not improve atherosclerotic to nonatherosclerotic lipoprotein levels.[52] Patients in the highest-risk groups are most likely to benefit from fibrate therapy if they are unable to achieve treatment goal with statin therapy and lifestyle modification (SOR A).

Table 7		
Secondary prevention guidelines		
Guideline	**Secondary Prevention**	**Qualifiers**
ACC/AHA	History of MI or stroke	None
AACE	Very high risk Extreme risk	Established CAD Progressive ASCVD including unstable angina after achieving LDL-C >70 mg/dL Established CAD in patients with diabetes, CKD stage 3 or greater, familial hypercholesterolemia History of premature ASCVD, men <55 and women <65

Data from Jellinger PS, Handelsman Y, Rosenblit PD, et al. American Association of Clinical Endocrinologists and American College of Endocrinology guidelines for management of dyslipidemia and prevention of cardiovascular disease. Endocr Pract 2017;23(Suppl 2):1–87; and Tonelli M, Muntner P, Lloyd A, et al. Risk of coronary events in people with chronic kidney disease compared with those with diabetes: a population-level cohort study. Lancet 2012;380(9844):807–14.

Table 8 Guideline based treatment goals	
Guideline	**Goal**
USPSTF	Low intensity <30% reduction in LDL-C
	Moderate intensity 30%–50% reduction in LDL-C
ACC/AHA	Moderate intensity 30%–50% reduction in LDL-C
	High intensity >50% reduction in LDL-C
AACE	Low risk: LDL-C <130 mg/dL, non-HLD-C <160 mg/dL
	Moderate risk: LDL-C <100 mg/dL, non-HDL-C <130 mg/dL
	High risk: LDL-C <100 mg/dL, non-HDL-C <130 mg/dL
	Very high risk: LDL-C <70 mg/dL, non-HDL-C <100 mg/dL
	Extreme risk: LDL-C <55 mg/dL, non-HDL-C <80 mg/dL

Data from Refs.[1,7,16,45]

Selective cholesterol absorption inhibitors

Selective cholesterol absorption inhibitors may be of use for primary and secondary prevention of cardiovascular events when added to a statin for patients with high ASCVD risk, CHD, or CHD risk equivalents. Ezetimibe is used as a second-line agent in risk reduction of ASCVD in primary and secondary prevention. Ezetimibe has demonstrated a reduction in low-density lipoprotein-cholesterol (LDL-C) from 12% to 19% when compared with placebo.[53] Use of this drug class in low-risk groups is unlikely to confer benefit (SOR B).

PCSK-9 inhibitors

PCSK-9 inhibitors are newly available monoclonal antibodies used for reduction of LDL-C. Two *Cochrane Reviews* looking at the use of PCSK-9 monoclonal antibodies in more than 20 trials showed a reduction in LDL-C between 30% and 54% with an absolute risk reduction of less than 1% for cardiovascular events.[50,54] Due primarily to high cost, routine use of PSCK-9 inhibitors for primary and secondary prevention of cardiovascular events is be limited (SOR A).

Cochrane Reviews

Cochrane Reviews have also been published on the use of niacin and B-complex vitamin for use in cardiovascular event reduction. There is no evidence that niacin or B-complex vitamins reduce deaths, MI, or stroke, or reduce mortality when used alone or with a statin.[55,56] Niacin or B-complex vitamins should not be used for prevention of cardiovascular events (SOR A).

Table 9 Drug class and expected low-density lipoprotein reduction			
Class	**Mechanism**	**Use**	**LDL-C Reduction**
Statins	HMG-CoA reductase	Primary and secondary prevention	Based on intensity (see **Table 8**)
Fibrates	Increase LDL catabolism through modulation of the LDL receptor/ligand interaction	Secondary	Minimal to no reduction in LDL-C
Ezetimibe	Blocks intestinal absorption	Secondary	12%–19% reduction in LDL-C
PCSK-9	Monoclonal antibodies	Secondary	30.2%–53.86% reduction in LDL-C

Data from Refs.[1,7,16,49–51,54]

For patients with stable CAD, established antianginal medications include β-blockers, calcium channel blockers, and long-acting nitrates. The ACC/AHA provides a class I recommendation for these medications in patients with stable CAD.[57] In such cases, optimal medical management has outcomes equal to or superior to revascularization alone. Patients on a single antianginal medication had lower combined mortality and MI. Patients on 2 antianginal medications had lower combined mortality, but higher rate of MI. Patients on 3 or more antianginal medications had similar rates of mortality and higher rates of MI than those on no antianginal medications.[57]

Ranolzaine (Ranexa)

Ranolzaine (Ranexa) is a newer antianginal agent that is typically added to an existing medication regimen. A *Cochrane Review* comparing ranolazine to placebo showed an uncertain effect on mortality and CVD when used as monotherapy or in combination therapy.[58] Patients on ranolazine also experienced higher rates of nonserious adverse events when compared with placebo.[57] There is some moderate-quality evidence that in patients with frequent angina attacks, ranolazine may decrease the number of angina episodes and improve quality of life when used as combination therapy (SOR C).[58]

Nonpharmacologic Strategies

Nonpharmacologic strategies for symptomatic CAD primarily include coronary artery bypass grafting and PCI that involve angioplasty and/or stenting. Patients receiving invasive treatments typically present to the emergency room with acute coronary syndromes and are managed according to existing protocols. A recent *Cochrane Review* evaluated invasive therapy versus conservative management for unstable angina and non-ST elevation MI. The review found that the patients who underwent PCI had lower rates of persistent chest pain, lower readmission rates, and decreased risk of MI over the next 3 to 5 years. They were, however, at increased risk of MI immediately following the procedure.[59] In patients with stable CAD deemed clinically to be at high risk for an ASCVD event, the ACC/AHA recommends the selective-invasive approach. Recommendations are based on which vessel is occluded (SOR C).

Patients with a recent cardiovascular event should routinely be referred to cardiac rehabilitation and offered psychological intervention (SOR A). These patients benefit both psychologically and physically from comprehensive cardiac rehabilitation programs following a cardiovascular event.[60,61] Cardiac rehabilitation decreases rates of hospitalization, but not the need for revascularization of nonfatal MI.[60] Patients with a history of MI who undergo psychological therapy have a reduction in cardiac mortality and psychological symptoms, including anxiety and depression.[61] Cardiac rehabilitation programs are time intensive and interdisciplinary and require effort by both providers and patients to optimize benefit.

Self-Management Strategies: The Key to Success

Working with patients to address modifiable risk factors is the most important aspect of CVD management. Modifiable risk factors include tobacco use, alcohol, and illicit drug use, overweight, poor dietary habits, and inadequate physical activity.[1,6,62] Smoking cessation decreases the risk greater for a cardiovascular event more than any pharmacologic intervention.[63] Dietary and physical activity recommendations are available to help providers and patients with realistic goal setting (**Table 10**).[1,49,62] The Mediterranean diet is of established benefit in patients with a

Table 10 Lifestyle recommendations based on guideline		
Guideline	Dietary Recommendations	Exercise Recommendations
USPSTF	Refer adults with risk of CVD for intensive behavioral counseling for dietary modification	Refer adults with risk of CVD for intensive behavioral counseling for exercise education
ACC/AHA	DASH dietary pattern Dietary intake that emphasizes vegetables, fruits, whole grains, low-fat dairy products, poultry, fish, legumes. Limit intake of sweets, sugar-sweetened beverages, and red meats	30–60 min of moderate-intensity aerobic activity at least 5 d a week, preferably 7 d a week
AACE	30 min of moderate-intensity physical activity (4-7 kcal/min) is recommend Can be met by single or multiple sessions of 10 min or more	More than 5 servings of fruits and vegetables a day, grains, fish, and lean meats

Data from Refs.[1,6,17,63]

history of a cardiovascular event.[64] Public health interventions in New York restricting trans saturated fats showed a significant reduction of both stroke and MI.[65,66]

SUMMARY

CAD is a leading international public health concern impacting quality-of-life global health expenditures. In-office therapy has traditionally focused on pharmacologic management of primary and secondary prevention. Primary prevention focuses on addressing known risk factors to prevent first cardiovascular events. Modifiable risk factors (see **Box 1**) should be regularly assessed in adults over the age of 20, even if they are thought to be free from ASCVD (SOR A).[17] Multiple clinical predictions models are available to help assess cardiovascular risk (see **Table 4**). Although external validation of these models is limited, they still offer the most systematic approach to risk assessment and their use is recommended (SOR A). Providers using the ACC/AHA calculator should be aware that this model likely overestimates risk.[21]

Lifestyle modifications are the cornerstone of CVD management (SOR A). They are also difficult to implement and maintain. Interventions such as smoking cessation, dietary modification, and efforts to increase physical activity have the most significant impact for both primary and secondary preventive efforts.

Patients with known CHD or having a CHD risk equivalent do not require screening. They require secondary prevention. Patients with recent or active chest pain require diagnostic testing rather than screening. Recommendations for the management of CAD risk vary among professional organizations (see **Table 6**).

Pharmacotherapy is beneficial in helping reduce primary and secondary cardiovascular events and is an important tool for reducing risk in the right patients. Intermediate- and low-risk patients do not require aggressive management, but higher-risk individuals do (SOR A). In patients greater than 75 years old, modifiable risk should be addressed and pharmacotherapy limited. For patients greater than 75 years old, initiation of statin therapy is not recommended for primary prevention. For patients in this age group already on statins, consider discontinuation if used for primary prevention (SOR A). There is minimal benefit for statin use in hypertensive patients aged 65 to 74 for primary prevention. Shared decision making should be used when considering initiating statin therapy in this patient population (SOR B). Dual pharmaco-therapy should be reserved for higher-risk individuals (SOR B). Some form of statin therapy is of benefit even if the patient has Statin intolerance and cannot tolerate high-dose statins (SOR B).

There is clear benefit for pharmacotherapy in secondary prevention with statins (SOR A). For patients who do not meet treatment goals based on AACE guidelines or expected LDL-C reduction on statin therapy, adding a fibrate or ezetimibe to their treatment regimen should be considered (SOR C). Adding further pharmacotherapy has not been shown to be of benefit in patients for primary or secondary cardiovascular event risk reduction in low-risk patients (SOR A).

REFERENCES

1. Jellinger PS, Handelsman Y, Rosenblit PD, et al. American Association of Clinical Endocrinologists and American College of Endocrinology guidelines for management of dyslipidemia and prevention of cardiovascular disease. Endocr Pract 2017;23(Suppl 2):1–87.
2. Mozaffarian D, Benjamin EJ, Go AS, et al. Heart disease and stroke statistics–2015 update: a report from the American Heart Association. Circulation 2015; 131(4):e29–322.
3. Coronary Artery Disease. Available at: http://www.clevelandclinicmeded.com/medicalpubs/diseasemanagement/cardiology/coronary-artery-disease/. Accessed July 31, 2017.
4. Rana JS, Liu JY, Moffet HH, et al. Diabetes and prior coronary heart disease are not necessarily risk equivalent for future coronary heart disease events. J Gen Intern Med 2016;31(4):387–93.
5. Expert Panel on Detection, Evaluation, and Treatment of High Blood Cholesterol in Adults. Executive summary of the third report of the National Cholesterol Education Program (NCEP) Expert Panel on Detection, Evaluation, and Treatment of High Blood Cholesterol in Adults (Adult Treatment Panel III). JAMA 2001;285(19):2486–97.
6. Eckel RH, Jakicic JM, Ard JD, et al. 2013 AHA/ACC guideline on lifestyle management to reduce cardiovascular risk: a report of the American College of Cardiology/American Heart Association Task Force on Practice Guidelines. Circulation 2014;129(25 Suppl 2):S76–99.
7. US Preventive Services Task Force, Bibbins-Domingo K, Grossman DC, Curry SJ, et al. Statin use for the primary prevention of cardiovascular disease in adults: US Preventive Services Task Force recommendation statement. JAMA 2016;316(19): 1997–2007.
8. Yusuf S, Hawken S, Ôunpuu S, et al. Effect of potentially modifiable risk factors associated with myocardial infarction in 52 countries (the INTERHEART study): case-control study. Lancet 2004;364(9438):937–52.
9. Kozor R, Grieve S, Bhindi R, et al. Cardiovascular impact of cocaine in regular asymptomatic users assessed by cardiovascular magnetic resonance imaging. Circulation 2012;126(Suppl 21):A18163.
10. Valtorta NK, Kanaan M, Gilbody S, et al. Loneliness and social isolation as risk factors for coronary heart disease and stroke: systematic review and meta-analysis of longitudinal observational studies. Heart 2016;102(13):1009–16.
11. Devitt M. Diagnosis of stable ischemic heart disease: recommendations from the ACP. Am Fam Physician 2013;88(7):469–70.
12. Menees DS, Bates ER. Evaluation of patients with suspected coronary artery disease. Coron Artery Dis 2010;21(7):386–90.

13. Carter CS, Servan-Schreiber D, Perlstein WM. Anxiety disorders and the syndrome of chest pain with normal coronary arteries: prevalence and pathophysiology. J Clin Psychiatry 1997;58(Suppl 3):70–3 [discussion: 74–5].
14. Qaseem A. Diagnosis of stable ischemic heart disease: summary of a clinical practice guideline from the American College of Physicians/American College of Cardiology Foundation/American Heart Association/American Association for Thoracic Surgery/Preventive Cardiovascular Nurses Association/Society of Thoracic Surgeons. Ann Intern Med 2012;157(10):729.
15. Loprinzi PD, Branscum A, Hanks J, et al. Healthy lifestyle characteristics and their joint association with cardiovascular disease biomarkers in US adults. Mayo Clin Proc 2016;91(4):432–42.
16. Strong JP, Malcom GT, McMahan CA, et al. Prevalence and extent of atherosclerosis in adolescents and young adults: implications for prevention from the pathobiological determinants of atherosclerosis in youth study. JAMA 1999;281(8):727–35.
17. Goff DC, Lloyd-Jones DM, Bennett G, et al. 2013 ACC/AHA guideline on the assessment of cardiovascular risk: a report of the American College of Cardiology/American Heart Association Task Force on Practice Guidelines. Circulation 2014;129(25 Suppl 2):S49–73.
18. Damen JAAG, Hooft L, Schuit E, et al. Prediction models for cardiovascular disease risk in the general population: systematic review. BMJ 2016;353:i2416.
19. Salisbury AC, Spertus JA. Realizing the potential of clinical risk prediction models: where are we now and what needs to change to better personalize delivery of care? Circ Cardiovasc Qual Outcomes 2015;8(4):332–4.
20. Berry JD, Liu K, Folsom AR, et al. Prevalence and progression of subclinical atherosclerosis in younger adults with low short-term but high lifetime estimated risk for cardiovascular disease: the coronary artery risk development in young adults study and multi-ethnic study of atherosclerosis. Circulation 2009;119(3): 382–9.
21. Rana JS, Tabada GH, Solomon MD, et al. Accuracy of the atherosclerotic cardiovascular risk equation in a large contemporary, multiethnic population. J Am Coll Cardiol 2016;67(18):2118–30.
22. Wessler BS, Lai Yh L, Kramer W, et al. Clinical prediction models for cardiovascular disease: Tufts Predictive Analytics and comparative effectiveness clinical prediction model database. Circ Cardiovasc Qual Outcomes 2015;8(4):368–75.
23. Pencina MJ, D'Agostino RB, Larson MG, et al. Predicting the 30-year risk of cardiovascular disease: the Framingham Heart Study. Circulation 2009;119(24): 3078–84.
24. Chou R, Arora B, Dana T, et al. Screening asymptomatic adults with resting or exercise electrocardiography: a review of the evidence for the U.S. Preventive Services Task Force. Ann Intern Med 2011;155(6):375.
25. Bulugahapitiya U, Siyambalapitiya S, Sithole J, et al. Is diabetes a coronary risk equivalent? Systematic review and meta-analysis. Diabet Med 2009;26(2):142–8.
26. Members WC, Greenland P, Alpert JS, et al. 2010 ACCF/AHA guideline for assessment of cardiovascular risk in asymptomatic adults: executive summary. Circulation 2010;122(25):2748–64.
27. Ärnlöv J, Evans JC, Meigs JB, et al. Low-grade albuminuria and incidence of cardiovascular disease events in nonhypertensive and nondiabetic individuals. Circulation 2005;112(7):969–75.
28. Ibsen H, Olsen MH, Wachtell K, et al. Reduction in albuminuria translates to reduction in cardiovascular events in hypertensive patients. Hypertension 2005; 45(2):198–202.

29. Bakris GL, Molitch M. Microalbuminuria as a risk predictor in diabetes: the continuing saga. Diabetes Care 2014;37(3):867–75.

30. Emerging Risk Factors Collaboration, Di Angelantonio E, Gao P, Pennells L, et al. Lipid-related markers and cardiovascular disease prediction. JAMA 2012; 307(23):2499–506.

31. Chang J, Paulson CP, Smith RF. Apolipoproteins for cardiovascular risk assessment. Am Fam Physician 2014;89(8). 662A-662B Online. Available at: http://www.aafp.org/afp/2014/0415/od2.html. Accessed August 28, 2017.

32. Sniderman AD, Williams K, Contois JH, et al. A meta-analysis of low-density lipoprotein cholesterol, non-high-density lipoprotein cholesterol, and apolipoprotein B as markers of cardiovascular risk. Circ Cardiovasc Qual Outcomes 2011; 4(3):337–45.

33. Verbeek R, Hovingh GK, Boekholdt SM. Non-high-density lipoprotein cholesterol: current status as cardiovascular marker. Curr Opin Lipidol 2015;26(6):502–10.

34. van Wijk DF, Boekholdt SM, Wareham NJ, et al. C-Reactive Protein, Fatal and Nonfatal Coronary Artery Disease, Stroke, and Peripheral Artery Disease in the Prospective EPIC-Norfolk Cohort Study. Arterioscler Thromb Vasc Biol 2013; 33(12):2888–94.

35. Cook NR, Paynter NP, Eaton CB, et al. Comparison of the Framingham and Reynolds Risk Scores for global cardiovascular risk prediction in the Multiethnic Women's Health Initiative. Circulation 2012;125(14):1748–56.

36. McClelland RL, Jorgensen NW, Budoff M, et al. 10-Year coronary heart disease risk prediction using coronary artery calcium and traditional risk factors: derivation in the MESA (Multi-Ethnic Study of Atherosclerosis) with validation in the HNR (Heinz Nixdorf Recall) study and the DHS (Dallas Heart Study). J Am Coll Cardiol 2015;66(15):1643–53.

37. Blaha MJ, Cainzos-Achirica M, Greenland P, et al. Role of coronary artery calcium score of zero and other negative risk markers for cardiovascular disease: the Multi-Ethnic Study of Atherosclerosis (MESA). Circulation 2016;133(9):849–58.

38. Angelantonio ED, Chowdhury R, Sarwar N, et al. B-type natriuretic peptides and cardiovascular risk. Circulation 2009;120(22):2177–87.

39. Sayols-Baixeras S, Lluís-Ganella C, Lucas G, et al. Pathogenesis of coronary artery disease: focus on genetic risk factors and identification of genetic variants. Appl Clin Genet 2014;7:15–32.

40. Nikpay M, Goel A, Won H-H, et al. A comprehensive 1000 genomes-based genome-wide association meta-analysis of coronary artery disease. Nat Genet 2015;47(10):1121–30.

41. Ruwanpathirana T, Owen A, Reid CM. Review on cardiovascular risk prediction. Cardiovasc Ther 2015;33(2):62–70.

42. Amarenco P, Steg PG. Stroke is a coronary heart disease risk equivalent: implications for future clinical trials in secondary stroke prevention. Eur Heart J 2008; 29(13):1605–7.

43. Touzé E, Varenne O, Chatellier G, et al. Risk of myocardial infarction and vascular death after transient ischemic attack and ischemic stroke: a systematic review and meta-analysis. Stroke 2005;36(12):2748–55.

44. Briasoulis A, Bakris GL. Chronic kidney disease as a coronary artery disease risk equivalent. Curr Cardiol Rep 2013;15(3):340.

45. Tonelli M, Muntner P, Lloyd A, et al. Risk of coronary events in people with chronic kidney disease compared with those with diabetes: a population-level cohort study. Lancet 2012;380(9844):807–14.

46. Bittencourt MS, Hulten E, Polonsky TS, et al. European Society of Cardiology-recommended coronary artery disease consortium pretest probability scores more accurately predict obstructive coronary disease and cardiovascular events than the Diamond and Forrester score: the Partners Registry. Circulation 2016; 134(3):201–11.

47. Pagidipati NJ, Navar AM, Mulder H, et al. Comparison of recommended eligibility for primary prevention statin therapy based on the US Preventive Services Task Force Recommendations vs the ACC/AHA guidelines. JAMA 2017;317(15):1563–7.

48. Mortensen MB, Nordestgaard BG, Afzal S, et al. ACC/AHA guidelines superior to ESC/EAS guidelines for primary prevention with statins in non-diabetic Europeans: the Copenhagen General Population Study. Eur Heart J 2017;38(8):586–94.

49. Fihn SD, Gardin JM, Abrams J, et al. 2012 ACCF/AHA/ACP/AATS/PCNA/SCAI/STS Guideline for the diagnosis and management of patients with stable ischemic heart disease: a report of the American College of Cardiology Foundation/American Heart Association Task Force on Practice Guidelines, and the American College of Physicians, American Association for Thoracic Surgery, Preventive Cardiovascular Nurses Association, Society for Cardiovascular Angiography and Interventions, and Society of Thoracic Surgeons. J Am Coll Cardiol 2012;60(24):e44–164.

50. Jakob T, Nordmann AJ, Schandelmaier S, et al. Fibrates for primary prevention of cardiovascular disease events. Cochrane Database Syst Rev 2016;(11):CD009753.

51. Wang D, Liu B, Tao W, et al. Fibrates for secondary prevention of cardiovascular disease and stroke. Cochrane Database Syst Rev 2015;(10):CD009580.

52. Chan SY, Mancini GBJ, Ignaszewski A, et al. Statins but not fibrates improve the atherogenic to anti-atherogenic lipoprotein particle ratio: a randomized crossover study. BMC Clin Pharmacol 2008;8:10.

53. Hammersley D, Signy M. Ezetimibe: an update on its clinical usefulness in specific patient groups. Ther Adv Chronic Dis 2017;8(1):4–11.

54. Schmidt AF, Pearce LS, Wilkins JT, et al. PCSK9 monoclonal antibodies for the primary and secondary prevention of cardiovascular disease. Cochrane Database Syst Rev 2017;(4):CD011748.

55. Niacin for primary and secondary prevention of cardiovascular events. PubMed - NCBI. Available at: https://www.ncbi.nlm.nih.gov/pubmed/?term=niacin+Schmandelmeir. Accessed July 31, 2017.

56. Martí-Carvajal AJ, Solà I, Lathyris D. Homocysteine-lowering interventions for preventing cardiovascular events. Cochrane Database Syst Rev 2015. https://doi.org/10.1002/14651858.CD006612.pub4. John Wiley & Sons, Ltd.

57. Kloner RA, Chaitman B. Angina and its management. J Cardiovasc Pharmacol Ther 2017;22(3):199–209.

58. Salazar CA, Basilio Flores JE, Veramendi Espinoza LE, et al. Ranolazine for stable angina pectoris. Cochrane Database Syst Rev 2017;(2):CD011747.

59. Fanning JP, Nyong J, Scott IA, et al. Routine invasive strategies versus selective invasive strategies for unstable angina and non-ST elevation myocardial infarction in the stent era. Cochrane Database Syst Rev 2016. https://doi.org/10.1002/14651858.CD004815.pub4. John Wiley & Sons, Ltd.

60. Anderson L, Brown JP, Clark AM, et al. Patient education in the management of coronary heart disease. Cochrane Database Syst Rev 2017. https://doi.org/10.1002/14651858.CD008895.pub3. John Wiley & Sons, Ltd.

61. Richards SH, Anderson L, Jenkinson CE, et al. Psychological interventions for coronary heart disease. Cochrane Database Syst Rev 2017. https://doi.org/10.1002/14651858.CD002902.pub4. John Wiley & Sons, Ltd.

62. US Preventive Services Task Force, Grossman DC, Bibbins-Domingo K, Curry SJ, et al. Behavioral counseling to promote a healthful diet and physical activity for cardiovascular disease prevention in adults without cardiovascular risk factors: US Preventive Services Task Force recommendation statement. JAMA 2017; 318(2):167–74.
63. Bakhru A, Erlinger TP. Smoking cessation and cardiovascular disease risk factors: results from the Third National Health and Nutrition Examination Survey. PLoS Med 2005;2(6). https://doi.org/10.1371/journal.pmed.0020160.
64. Mediterranean Diet Improves High-Density Lipoprotein Function in High-Cardiovascular-Risk Individuals. Clinical Perspective. Circulation. Available at: http://circ.ahajournals.org/content/135/7/633?download=true. Accessed July 31, 2017.
65. Brandt EJ, Myerson R, Perraillon MC, et al. Hospital admissions for myocardial infarction and stroke before and after the trans-fatty acid restrictions in New York. JAMA Cardiol 2017;2(6):627–34.
66. Monguchi T, Hara T, Hasokawa M, et al. Excessive intake of trans fatty acid accelerates atherosclerosis through promoting inflammation and oxidative stress in a mouse model of hyperlipidemia. J Cardiol 2017;70(2):121–7.
67. D'Agostino RB, Vasan RS, Pencina MJ, et al. General cardiovascular risk profile for use in primary care: the Framingham Heart Study. Circulation 2008;117(6): 743–53.
68. Ridker PM, Buring JE, Rifai N, et al. Development and validation of improved algorithms for the assessment of global cardiovascular risk in women: the Reynolds Risk Score. JAMA 2007;297(6):611–9.
69. Goff DC, Lloyd-Jones DM, Bennett G, et al. American College of Cardiology/American Heart Association Task Force on Practice Guidelines. 2013 ACC/AHA guideline on the assessment of cardiovascular risk: a report of the American College of Cardiology/American Heart Association Task Force on Practice Guidelines. Circulation 2014;129(25 Suppl 2):S49–73.
70. Budoff MJ, McClelland RL, Nasir K, et al. Cardiovascular events with absent or minimal coronary calcification: the Multi-Ethnic Study of Atherosclerosis (MESA). American Heart Journal 2009;158(4):554–61.
71. Amarenco P, Steg PG. Stroke is a coronary heart disease risk equivalent: implications for future clinical trials in secondary stroke prevention. European Heart Journal 2008;29(13):1605–7.
72. Touzé E, Varenne O, Chatellier G, et al. Risk of myocardial infarction and vascular death after transient ischemic attack and ischemic stroke: a systematic review and meta-analysis. Stroke 2005;36(12):2748–55.
73. Rana JS, Liu JY, Moffet HH, et al. Diabetes and Prior Coronary Heart Disease are Not Necessarily Risk Equivalent for Future Coronary Heart Disease Events. Journal of General Internal Medicine 2016;1(4):387–93.

Heart Failure
Optimizing Recognition and
Management in Outpatient Settings

Brian E. Neubauer, MD[a,b,*], Jeffery T. Gray, MD[c],
Brian A. Hemann, MD[a,d]

KEYWORDS

- Heart failure • Guideline-directed care • Management • Self-care

KEY POINTS

- Heart failure is a complex clinical syndrome associated with a range of clinical signs and symptoms and results from a wide variety of underlying causes.
- The prevalence of heart failure is expected to grow significantly in the United States over the next several decades representing a significant health challenge.
- As a major chronic disease, heart failure care is a dominant driver of health expenses.
- In order to make the strongest impact in the face of these challenges, primary care clinicians must recognize patients with risk factors and structural heart conditions in order to institute prevention and early evidence-based care measures.

INTRODUCTION

Heart failure (HF) is a complex and heterogeneous clinical syndrome associated with a range of clinical signs and symptoms resulting from a wide variety of underlying causes. Given its complexity, HF has generally been viewed as a syndrome defined in the following way (**Box 1**).

Disclosure Statement: The views expressed in this article are those of the authors and do not necessarily reflect the official policy or position of the Uniformed Services University of the Health Sciences, Walter Reed National Military Medical Center, the United States Air Force, Army, Navy, Department of Defense, or the US government.
[a] Department of Medicine, Uniformed Services University of the Health Sciences, 4301 Jones Bridge Road, Bethesda, MD 20889, USA; [b] Department of Medicine, Walter Reed National Military Medical Center, 8901 Wisconsin Avenue, Bethesda, MD 20889, USA; [c] Internal Medicine Residency, Department of Medicine, Walter Reed National Military Medical Center, 8901 Wisconsin Avenue, Bethesda, MD 20889-5600, USA; [d] Walter Reed National Military Medical Center, 8901 Wisconsin Avenue, Bethesda, MD 20889-5600, USA
* Corresponding author. Uniformed Services University, MED-EDP, Building 53, Room 53, 4301 Jones Bridge Road, Bethesda, MD 20814.
E-mail address: Brian.neubauer@usuhs.edu

> **Box 1**
> **Definition of heart failure as a syndrome**
>
> HF is a complex clinical syndrome
> - Characterized by a variety of typical symptoms and signs (see **Table 1**)
> - Develops as a consequence of a wide variety of causes
> - That results in structural and functional impairments of either systolic and/or diastolic function of the heart leading to a reduced cardiac output and/or elevated filling pressures
> - Typically chronic and progressive in nature
>
> *Data from* Refs.[1–3]

Nature of the Problem

HF represents a significant and multifaceted challenge for patients, health care providers and systems, managed care organizations, and governments. Epidemiologically, HF is a common chronic medical condition with an annual incidence of approximately 915,000 cases per year.[4,5] HF impacts approximately 5.7 million adult Americans.[5] As the US population ages and mortality rates decline as a result of improved care, the prevalence of HF is projected to increase 46% from 2012 to 2030.[5] This increase has important implications because HF is a major contributor to mortality, listed as the primary cause of approximately 2.5% of all deaths and as a contributing factor in up to 12.0% of deaths.[5] HF also places significant economic demands on health systems with estimated overall costs ranging from $30.7 and $127.0 billion annually.[6,7] If these costs continue as projected, by the year 2030, $244 to $443 will be spent on HF care for every US adult.[6,7] Care relating to HF is responsible for approximately 1.75 million office visits and more than 0.5 million emergency department visits annually.[5] Given an anticipated physician shortfall[8] and disparities in specialty care across geographic regions,[9] the health care community must work together to incorporate evidence-based prevention and treatment strategies to meet the anticipated challenges that lie ahead.

MANAGEMENT
Diagnosis of Heart Failure

To improve HF outcomes, clinicians should emphasize prevention in patients at risk of HF and promptly diagnose and treat patients with overt HF. HF is staged using the American College of Cardiology Foundation (ACCF)/American Heart Association's (AHA) stages of HF classification scheme (**Fig. 1**).[10] This staging system has additional value for prognostication, as studies have demonstrated a decreased 5-year survival at progressive stages (stage A, 97%; stage B, 96%; stage C, 75%; stage D, 20%).[11]

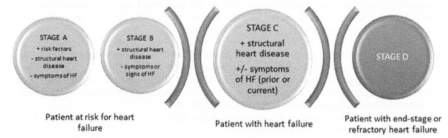

Fig. 1. The ACCF/AHA's stages of heart failure. (*Data from* Yancy CW, Jessup M, Bozkurt B, et al. 2013 ACCF/AHA guideline for the management of heart failure: executive summary: a report of the American College of Cardiology Foundation/American Heart Association Task Force on Practice guidelines. Circulation 2013;128(16):1810–52.)

To optimize HF, the commonly used secondary-tertiary prevention care model[12] must be flipped to promote primary prevention by explicitly incorporating a strategy for the assessment and management of the risk factors for HF and recognition of structural heart disease in daily practice.

The traditional risk factors for HF include coronary heart disease, hypertension, tobacco use (current and past smokers), obesity, and diabetes mellitus.[13] There is a variety of other risk factors, including family history of cardiomyopathy; history of endocrine disease; obstructive sleep apnea; metabolic syndrome; significant use of alcohol, cocaine, or amphetamines; prior chemotherapy use (eg, anthracyclines); history of living or spending significant time in Mexico or Central or South America (areas endemic for Chagas disease); and arrhythmias.[1] When risk factors are identified, clinicians should assess the symptoms and signs of HF, consider screening for structural heart disease, and implement risk factor modification. In this context, structural heart disease refers to congenital or valvular heart disease, structural cardiac changes, such as left ventricular (LV) hypertrophy, asymptomatic LV systolic and/or diastolic dysfunction, and geometric chamber distortion.[14]

Patients with HF can present with a variety of symptoms and signs, which may complicate rapid and reliable recognition of this diagnosis. These findings are reviewed in **Table 1**.

Several diagnostic strategies are helpful for the recognition and diagnosis of HF. These strategies include the Framingham criteria[18] (**Table 2**), the Boston criteria,[19] and the European Society of Cardiology criteria.[1] Each of these approaches uses a combination of symptoms, physical examination findings, and chest radiologic features that are readily available in the primary care setting. Although the utility of these tools is generally similar at the point of care,[20] the Framingham criteria are currently recommended by the Institute for Clinical Systems Improvement.[21]

In addition to the history, physical examination, and chest radiograph, an electrocardiogram (ECG) should routinely be obtained as part of the evaluation in patients with HF. Although there are no ECG findings that are highly specific for HF, the presence of LV or right ventricular hypertrophy, atrial or ventricular arrhythmias, atrioventricular and intraventricular conduction blocks and evidence of myocardial infarction (MI) and left and/or right atrial abnormalities support the diagnosis.[22]

For patients with suspected HF based on these initial steps, natriuretic peptides (NPs), such as N-terminal pro b-type natriuretic peptide (NT-proBNP) or BNP, can

Table 1 Typical symptoms and signs of heart failure	
Symptoms	**Signs**
Dyspnea[a]	Elevated jugular venous pressure[a]
Orthopnea[a]	Positive abdomino-jugular reflux[a]
Paroxysmal nocturnal dyspnea[a]	S3[a]
Fatigue[a]	Laterally displaced apical impulse[a]
Lower extremity edema[a]	Pulmonary rales[a]
Reduced exercise tolerance[a]	Peripheral edema (lower extremities, scrotum,
Cough, particularly nocturnal	sacrum)[a]
Wheezing	Tachycardia[a]
Bendopnea[15] or kamptapnea[16] (dyspnea	Narrow pulse pressure[a]
associated with bending forward)	Dullness to percussion, decreased breath sounds at
	bases of lungs (indicates pleural effusion)
	Weight gain

[a] Most common or most typical findings on history and physical exam.
Data from Refs.[1,3,17]

Table 2
Framingham heart failure diagnostic criteria

Diagnosis of HF Requires the Simultaneous Presence of at Least 2 Major Criteria or 1 Major and 2 Minor Criteria

Major Criteria	Minor Criteria[a]
Paroxysmal nocturnal dyspnea	Bilateral ankle edema
Neck vein distention	Nocturnal cough
Rales	Dyspnea on ordinary exertion
Radiographic cardiomegaly	Hepatomegaly
Acute pulmonary edema	Pleural effusion
S3	Decrease in vital capacity by one-third from maximum recorded
Increased central venous pressure (>16 cm H_2O at right atrium)	Tachycardia (>120 beats per minute)
Hepatojugular reflux	
Weight loss >4.5 kg in 5 d in response to treatment	

[a] Minor criteria are only acceptable if they cannot be attributed to another medical condition (eg, pulmonary hypertension, chronic lung disease, cirrhosis, ascites, or the nephrotic syndrome).

Data from McKee PA, Castelli WP, McNamara PM, et al. The natural history of congestive heart failure: the Framingham study. N Engl J Med 1971;285(26):1442.

help provide additional diagnostic value. NPs are readily available, provide high negative predictive values (useful for ruling out HF), and have good prognostic value.[23] NPs can also be useful to rule in the diagnosis of HF if clinicians are mindful that the clinical setting (pretest probability), specific cut points, and patient characteristics all impact the interpretation of NP values. In the outpatient, nonacute setting, the cutoff point for BNP is 35 pg/mL and 125 pg/mL for NT-proBNP.[1]

If elevated NP levels support the diagnosis of HF, patients should be referred for evaluation of cardiac structure and function (specifically LV ejection fraction [LVEF]). This evaluation is typically done using transthoracic echocardiography, which is widely available and relatively inexpensive.

As part of the diagnostic evaluation, clinicians should determine the stage of HF using the ACCF/AHA's system. For patients with stage A or B HF, the emphasis should be on risk factor modification and treatment of structural heart conditions. For patients with stage B HF, further stratification with echocardiography to detect the presence of systolic or diastolic dysfunction is helpful to direct therapy and predict the risk of progression to stage C and D. Traditionally, this classification was based on LVEF and split into systolic HF (HF with reduced EF [HFrEF]) and diastolic HF (HF with preserved EF [HFpEF]). Current use of LVEF as the determinant criteria proposes an LVEF greater than 50% signifying HFpEF and an LVEF less than 40% denoting HFrEF. Patients with an LVEF between 40% and 49%, HF with midrange EF, occupy an area of uncertainty in the literature.[1] Defining the stage of HF is important for directing specific management.

TREATMENT
Stage A

Risk factor identification and management is key for patients in stage A (**Fig. 2, Table 3**). The goal is to prevent progression to more advanced stages of HF.

Hypertension

Multiple studies illustrate the link between poorly controlled hypertension and the development of HF.[24,25] Strict blood pressure control is emphasized in the

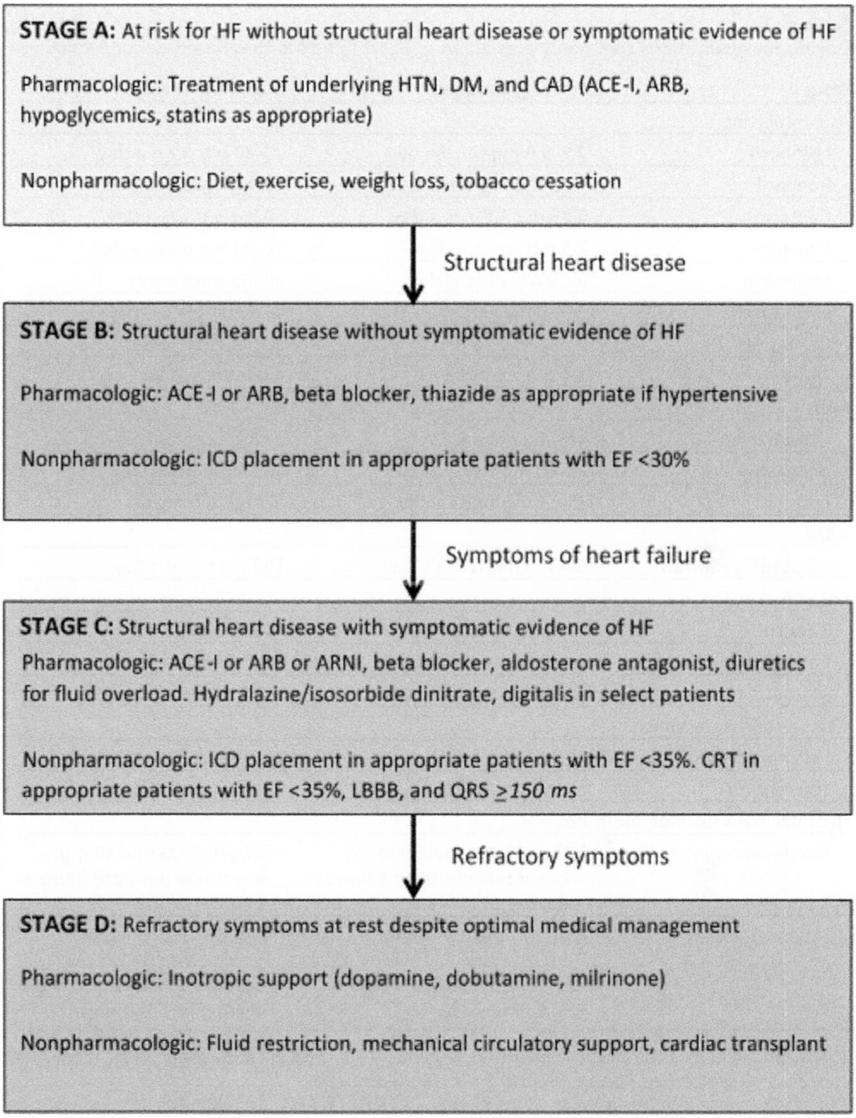

STAGE A: At risk for HF without structural heart disease or symptomatic evidence of HF

Pharmacologic: Treatment of underlying HTN, DM, and CAD (ACE-I, ARB, hypoglycemics, statins as appropriate)

Nonpharmacologic: Diet, exercise, weight loss, tobacco cessation

Structural heart disease

STAGE B: Structural heart disease without symptomatic evidence of HF

Pharmacologic: ACE-I or ARB, beta blocker, thiazide as appropriate if hypertensive

Nonpharmacologic: ICD placement in appropriate patients with EF <30%

Symptoms of heart failure

STAGE C: Structural heart disease with symptomatic evidence of HF
Pharmacologic: ACE-I or ARB or ARNI, beta blocker, aldosterone antagonist, diuretics for fluid overload. Hydralazine/isosorbide dinitrate, digitalis in select patients

Nonpharmacologic: ICD placement in appropriate patients with EF <35%. CRT in appropriate patients with EF <35%, LBBB, and QRS ≥150 ms

Refractory symptoms

STAGE D: Refractory symptoms at rest despite optimal medical management

Pharmacologic: Inotropic support (dopamine, dobutamine, milrinone)

Nonpharmacologic: Fluid restriction, mechanical circulatory support, cardiac transplant

Fig. 2. Treatment of HF by stage. ACE-I, angiotensin-converting enzyme inhibitors; ARB, angiotensin-receptor blocker; ARNI, angiotensin receptor/neprilysin inhibitor; CAD, coronary artery disease; CRT, cardiac resynchronization therapy; DM, diabetes mellitus; HTN, hypertension; ICD, implantable cardioverter-defibrillator; LBBB, left bundle branch block.

American College of Cardiology (ACC)/AHA/Heart Failure Society of America's (HFSA) 2017 update to the 2013 guidelines.[26] For patients with stage A HF and underlying hypertension, blood pressure should be controlled to a goal of less than 130/80 mm Hg.[26] In patients with hypertensive heart disease, echocardiography helps determine cardiac function.[27] If structural heart disease is noted, patients are placed in stage B.

Table 3
Dosing for medications commonly prescribed in heart failure with reduced ejection fraction

Drug	Starting Dosage	Maximum Dosage
ACE inhibitors		
Lisinopril	2.5–5.0 mg once a day	20–40 mg once a day
Ramipril	1.25–2.5 mg once a day	10 mg once a day
Captopril	6.25 mg 3 times a day	50 mg 3 times a day
Enalapril	2.5 mg twice a day	10–20 mg twice a day
Fosinopril	5–10 mg once a day	40 mg once a day
Perindopril	2 mg once a day	8–16 mg once a day
Quinapril	5 mg twice a day	20 mg twice a day
Trandolapril	1 mg once a day	4 mg once a day
ARBs		
Candesartan	4–8 mg once a day	32 mg once a day
Valsartan	20–40 mg twice a day	160 mg twice a day
Losartan	25–50 mg once a day	50–150 mg once a day
ARNI		
Sacubitril/valsartan	50–100 mg twice a day	200 mg twice a day
Beta-blockers		
Bisoprolol	1.25 mg once a day	10 mg once a day
Carvedilol	3.125 mg twice a day	50 mg twice a day
Metoprolol succinate ER	12.5–25.0 mg once a day	200 mg once a day
Aldosterone antagonists		
Spironolactone	12.5–25.0 mg once a day	25 mg once or twice a day
Eplerenone	25 mg once a day	50 mg once a day
Hydralazine/isosorbide dinitrate		
Fixed-dose combination	37.5 mg hydralazine/20 mg isosorbide dinitrate 3 times a day	75 mg hydralazine/40 mg isosorbide dinitrate 3 times a day
Separate dosing	Hydralazine: 25–50 mg 3–4 times a day Isosorbide dinitrate: 20–30 mg 3–4 times a day	Hydralazine: 300 mg/d divided into 3–4 doses Isosorbide dinitrate: 120 mg/d divided into 3–4 doses

Abbreviations: ACE, angiotensin-converting enzyme; ARB, angiotensin-receptor blocker; ARNI, angiotensin receptor/neprilysin inhibitor; ER, extended release.

Data from Yancy CW, Jessup M, Bozkurt B, et al. 2013 ACCF/AHA guideline for the management of heart failure: executive summary: a report of the American College of Cardiology Foundation/ American Heart Association Task Force on practice guidelines. Circulation 2013;128(16):1810–52.

Hyperlipidemia

Because of the inherit link between atherosclerosis and ischemic cardiomyopathy, the treatment of at-risk patients with statin therapy is recommended to decrease the long-term cardiovascular risk.[28]

Diabetes mellitus

Poor glycemic control greatly increases the risk of developing HF. Patients with uncontrolled diabetes (hemoglobin A1c [HgbA1c] >10.5%) are several-fold more likely to develop HF compared with those who have a normal HgbA1c (<6.5%).[29] Women with diabetes may be at particular risk.[30] In diabetic patients, the use of an angiotensin-converting enzyme (ACE) inhibitor or an angiotensin-receptor blocker (ARB) reduces HF risk.[31] Adequate glycemic control lowers the cardiovascular risk and decreases the risk of HF progression.

Coronary artery disease
Atherosclerotic disease is also strongly associated with the development of HF. Treatment of at-risk patients with a statin and ACE inhibitor can lower the risk of progression to HF.[32,33]

Tobacco
Tobacco use is a well-defined risk factor for the development of HF, so smoking cessation is a key component of treatment.[34]

Obesity
Obesity has also been shown to increase HF risk. Therefore, educating patients on the importance of diet, exercise, and weight loss is an essential role of the primary care clinician in reducing progression to structural or symptomatic HF.

Stage B

Risk factor management applies to patients with all stages of HF, including stage B. Patients with asymptomatic reduced LVEF are at risk of increased mortality compared with those with normal LVEF.[35,36] Certain medications and interventions in asymptomatic patients with decreased EF or LV hypertrophy have established benefits in terms of morbidity and mortality. This section discusses pharmacologic and nonpharmacologic treatment options for patients with stage B HF.

Pharmacologic treatments
Angiotensin-converting enzyme inhibitors These medications block ACE and subsequently inhibit the negative myocardial remodeling effects elicited by the renin-angiotensin system. They have been widely studied and show significant benefit in preventing symptomatic HF in patients with a reduced EF, with or without preceding MI. One study showed that the use of enalapril for 3 years improved hospitalization rates and long-term survival up to 12 years in patients with LV systolic dysfunction in both symptomatic and asymptomatic patients.[37] Many ACE inhibitors have been studied, including enalapril, captopril, ramipril, and lisinopril, all of which have been shown to be effective.[38] If tolerated, an ACE inhibitor should be initiated in any patient with evidence of reduced EF on echocardiography. The side effects of ACE inhibitors include cough, angioedema, hypotension, and hyperkalemia.

Angiotensin-receptor blockers Although not as well studied as ACE inhibitors, ARBs are widely accepted as an alternative to ACE inhibitors to prevent progression to stage C HF. A 2003 trial showed that valsartan was noninferior to captopril in reducing cardiovascular outcomes after MI in patients with reduced LVEF.[39] In particular, ARBs are an option in those patients who are intolerant of ACE inhibitors because of cough or angioedema. Like ACE inhibitors, ARBs should be used with caution in patients at risk for hypotension, renal dysfunction, or hyperkalemia.[39] Combination treatment with an ACE inhibitor and an ARB has been associated with *increased* rates of adverse events without a clear benefit, so these two classes of medications should not be used in combination.[39]

Beta-blockers Similar to ACE inhibitors and ARBs, beta-blockers reduce strain on the heart and subsequently lower maladaptive LV remodeling. Three beta-blockers have been shown to improve mortality in patients with HF: metoprolol succinate, carvedilol, and bisoprolol.[40–42] The ACCF/AHA's 2013 guidelines give a class I recommendation for the use of these beta-blockers in any patient with a reduced EF, although the supporting evidence is stronger in those patients with a previous MI.[3] Potential side effects of beta-blockers include hypotension, fatigue, heart block, and fluid retention. They should also be used with caution in patients with underlying symptomatic bradycardia or severe reactive airway disease.

Thiazide diuretics Treatment of underlying hypertension is essential to prevent progression to symptomatic HF. The Antihypertensive and Lipid-Lowering Treatment to Prevent Heart Attack Trial (ALLHAT) demonstrated the benefit of thiazide diuretics in preventing HF in hypertensive patients.[43] Although chlorthalidone was studied in the ALLHAT trial, other thiazide diuretics are reasonable options. The side effects of thiazide diuretics include hypotension, hyperuricemia, and various electrolyte derangements.

Calcium channel blockers These medications may cause harm because of their negative inotropic effects and tendency to lead to fluid retention and should generally be avoided in patients with a low EF.[3] If calcium channel blockers are needed to help manage refractory hypertension in patients with HF, amlodipine and felodipine are preferred, as they have been shown not to increase mortality in HF.[44]

Nonpharmacologic treatments

Implantable cardiac defibrillator Patients with a prior MI and reduced EF are at risk for fatal arrhythmias. One trial demonstrated that implantation of an implantable cardiac defibrillator (ICD) in combination with medical therapy in post-MI patients with an EF less than 30% improved mortality at 20 months compared with medical therapy alone, regardless of New York Heart Association (NYHA) class.[45] The 2013 ACCF/AHA's HF guidelines consider ICD implantation if patients meet the following inclusion criteria: stage B HF, at least 40 days after MI, LVEF of 30% or less, and on guideline-directed medical therapy.[3]

Stage C

Stage C HF refers to those with evidence of structural heart disease and symptoms of HF. This section highlights that treatment of HF is constantly evolving, and studies in recent years have led to novel treatment options. Additionally, the ACC/AHA/HFSA's 2017 update to the ACCF/AHA's 2013 HF guidelines emphasizes blood pressure control in patients with stage C HFrEF and underlying hypertension.[26] In these patients, the medications discussed later should ideally be titrated until the systolic blood pressure is less than 130 mm Hg.[26]

Pharmacologic treatments

Angiotensin-converting enzyme inhibitors ACE inhibitors improve mortality in patients with HFrEF and should be prescribed to all patients with stage C HF unless otherwise contraindicated. Contraindications include pregnancy, history of angioedema, and renal failure. The mortality benefit is a class effect, so any ACE inhibitor can be used. Lisinopril or ramipril are good first options because of the simplicity (once daily) of dosing. Initiate ACE inhibitors at low doses and titrate to the goal as tolerated (see **Table 3**). Renal function and potassium levels should be monitored periodically.

Angiotensin-receptor blockers ARBs are a good option for patients who are intolerant of ACE inhibitors, particularly those with cough. They are also reasonable in patients who have angioedema while on an ACE inhibitor, although ARBs have also been associated with angioedema; caution is advised if switching for this indication.[46] Start ARBs at low doses and titrate slowly to the goal (see **Table 3**). With the exception of cough and angioedema, the adverse effects are similar to those for ACE inhibitors.

Angiotensin receptor/neprilysin inhibitor The Angiotensin-Neprilysin Inhibition versus Enalapril in Heart Failure (PARADIGM-HF) trial changed the treatment of stage C HF. This study randomized patients with NYHA II to IV HFrEF to enalapril or a combination of valsartan and sacubitril, a neprilysin inhibitor.[47] Neprilysin degrades vasoactive peptides, including natriuretic peptides and adrenomedullin, inhibiting sodium retention and maladaptive remodeling.[47] The trial was stopped early, as sacubitril/valsartan was associated with lower rates of death from cardiovascular causes, increased time to the first hospitalization for HF, and improved symptoms.[47] In terms of adverse effects, the angiotensin receptor/neprilysin inhibitor (ARNI) was associated with higher rates of hypotension and angioedema when compared with enalapril but lower rates of renal impairment, hyperkalemia, and cough.[47] ARNIs are contraindicated in patients with a history of angioedema.[26] The 2017 update to the 2013 ACCF/AHA guidelines recommend *switching* to the ARNI in patients with chronic, symptomatic HFrEF who have tolerated an ACE inhibitor or an ARB.[26] In patients who cannot tolerate an ARNI, or for whom the medication is cost prohibitive, continued use of an ACE inhibitor or ARB is strongly recommended.[26] An ARNI should never be administered with an ACE inhibitor, and a 36-hour washout period is necessary before switching from or to an ACE inhibitor.[48]

The dosing of sacubitril/valsartan is not as straightforward as that for ACE inhibitors or ARBs. Currently, there are 3 sacubitril/valsartan dosing formulations available. These formulations are 24/26 mg, 49/51 mg, and 97/103 mg, having respective total doses of 50 mg, 100 mg, and 200 mg.

- In patients at a goal dosage of an ACE inhibitor or ARB (>10 mg/d of enalapril or greater than 160 mg/d of valsartan or equivalent), the starting dosage is 100 mg (49/51) twice daily. This dosage should be doubled to 200 mg (97/103) twice daily in 2 to 4 weeks as tolerated.[48]
- In patients previously on a low-dose ACE inhibitor or ARB, the starting dosage is 50 mg (24/26) twice daily. It should be noted that this dosage was not studied in the trial. The dosage should be doubled to 100 mg (49/51) twice daily in 2 to 4 weeks as tolerated.[48]

Beta-blockers Three beta-blockers have been shown to reduce the risk of death in patients with HF: bisoprolol, carvedilol, and sustained-released metoprolol succinate.[40–42] Bisoprolol is not typically available in the United States. An approved beta-blocker should be initiated in all patients with reduced EF; providers should not wait until an ACE inhibitor, ARB, or ARNI is titrated to the goal dose before starting a beta-blocker. The Carvedilol or Metoprolol European Trial (COMET) demonstrated improved all-cause mortality with carvedilol compared with short-acting metoprolol tartrate.[49] Metoprolol succinate has less of a blood pressure effect than carvedilol and may be a better choice in patients in whom dosing is limited by hypotension.

Like ACE inhibitors or ARBs, beta-blockers should be started at low doses (see **Table 3**) and titrated very slowly to ensure they are tolerated. Beta-blockers should be used with caution in patients with a history of asymptomatic bradycardia or reactive airway disease. They can also lead to worsening fluid retention, fatigue, heart block, and/or hypotension. Fluid retention should be managed with diuretics, and the dose of beta-blocker should be reduced if bradycardia is accompanied by symptoms or a high-degree heart block.[3]

Aldosterone antagonists Spironolactone and eplerenone improve mortality and hospitalization rates in select patients with stage C HF, particularly patients with NYHA class III to IV HFrEF already on an ACE inhibitor or ARB and a beta-blocker. They are also recommended in patients with NYHA class II HFrEF and a prior cardiovascular hospitalization.[3] In the Randomized Aldactone Evaluation Study (RALES), spironolactone use reduced all-course mortality and hospitalization rates in patients with chronic HFrEF and LVEF less than 35%.[50] Similarly, eplerenone reduced all-cause deaths and HF hospitalizations in patients with NYHA class II to IV symptoms and reduced EF ($\leq$30% or 35% and QRS >130 ms on ECG).[51] Because of the risk of life-threatening hyperkalemia, proper patient selection is essential for these medications. Aldosterone antagonists should not be started in men with creatinine greater than 2.5 mg/dL, women with creatinine greater than 2.0 mg/dL, or any patient with a serum potassium of 5.0 mEq/L or greater or history of severe hyperkalemia.[3] Potassium levels greater than 5.5 mEq/L while on an aldosterone antagonist should trigger discontinuation or dose reduction of the drug. Although eplerenone is more expensive than spironolactone, it has a significantly lower risk of gynecomastia and can be used in patients who develop this side effect on spironolactone.

Hydralazine and isosorbide dinitrate This combination is recommended for self-described African American patients with NYHA class III to IV HFrEF despite optimal medical therapy.[3,52] The starting dosage of this combination is 37.5 mg of hydralazine hydrochloride and 20 mg of isosorbide dinitrate 3 times daily (see **Table 3**), which can be titrated as tolerated to 2 tablets 3 times a day. Adverse effects include headache, dizziness, and gastrointestinal upset; compliance rates may be low because of the dosing regimen.

Loop diuretics Loop diuretics are preferred to improve fluid retention in patients with HF. Furosemide is the most widely used loop diuretic. Dosing should start low and be adjusted with the goal of clinical euvolemia. Measurement of daily weights is one simple way to ensure adequate diuresis. Diuresis should be accompanied by dietary sodium restriction in order to prevent diuretic resistance (see Self-Management). In general, discontinue thiazide diuretics before the initiation of a loop diuretic. In some cases, patients may develop a syndrome of diuretic resistance requiring alternative strategies, such as concomitant use of acetazolamide or a thiazide diuretic as sequential nephron blockade.[53] These patients should generally be comanaged with a cardiologist.

Ivabradine Similar to sacubitril/valsartan, ivabradine is another new therapeutic option in the treatment of stage C HFrEF. Ivabradine selectively inhibits the funny current (I_f) in the sinoatrial node to lower the heart rate.[54] It reduces hospitalization rates but not mortality.[55] It is recommended in patients with NYHA class II to III HFrEF with an LVEF of 35% or less and a heart rate in sinus rhythm 70 or greater beats per minute at rest despite maximum-dose beta blockade.[26]

Digoxin Digoxin may be considered in patients with persistent symptoms despite maximal medical management. Digoxin improves hospitalization rates and symptoms but not mortality.[56] Digoxin is started at a dosage of 0.125 to 0.25 mg daily and does not need a loading dose if used for the treatment of HF. It is typically well tolerated at low plasma levels (0.5–0.9 ng/mL) but can have major toxic effects if not dosed properly, especially in elderly patients. Toxicity includes serious cardiac arrhythmias, gastrointestinal symptoms, visual disturbances, and confusion. Because of its effect on the atrioventricular node, digoxin should be used with caution in patients on beta-blocker therapy.

Nonpharmacologic treatments
Dietary sodium and fluid restriction are essential nonpharmacologic interventions in the treatment of HF. These interventions are discussed in the Self-care section.

Implantable cardiac defibrillator In patients with symptomatic HF, ICD placement has been shown to reduce 5-year mortality in patients with symptomatic HF and an LVEF of 35% or less.[57] Only consider ICD placement if the LVEF remains at 35% or less on 3 to 6 months of optimal medical therapy, as ventricular function may improve at greater than this cutoff with optimal medical management.[3] ICDs are indicated only for patients with good functional status and should not be placed in patients with NYHA class IV disease (unless the patients are ambulatory) or in patients whose life expectancy is less than 1 year.[3]

Cardiac resynchronization therapy Also known as biventricular pacing, cardiac resynchronization therapy (CRT) refers to the simultaneous pacing of both ventricles. CRT improves ventricular contraction and helps reverse ventricular remodeling. Additionally, CRT can increase blood pressure and allow for titration of other medications toward goal dosing.[3] CRT has a class I recommendation in patients with NYHA class II, III, or ambulatory IV symptoms on medical management with an LVEF of 35% or less, sinus rhythm, and a left bundle branch block (LBBB) with a QRS of 150 ms or greater.[3] CRT can also be considered in select patients with a non-LBBB or in those with a QRS of 120 to 149 ms.

Stage D

Stage D HF, also known as advanced or refractory disease, refers to the presence of severe symptoms despite maximum medical therapy. End-stage HF has a very high mortality rate of approximately 75% at 1 year, so it is important to ensure accurate staging.[58] Before confirming stage D HF, it is important to fully exclude other underlying conditions (such as thyroid or chronic lung diseases) and verify that medication noncompliance or inadequate sodium restriction are not contributing to persistent symptoms.[59,60] There are various advanced and specialized treatment options for stage D HF, including positive inotropes (eg, dobutamine and milrinone), mechanical circulatory support with ventricular assist devices, and cardiac transplantation (in eligible patients) available for advanced HF. The prognosis is poor, and goals of care should be discussed with patients when considering these options. The medical management of stage D HF is generally guided by a HF specialist. From a team-based care perspective, goals of care and end-of-life discussions are essential in end-stage disease; primary care physicians are well suited to engage in these conversations and should include palliative care specialists when appropriate.[3,61,62]

Heart Failure with Preserved Ejection Fraction

HFpEF refers to impaired filling of the LV with a normal EF. The treatment of HFpEF focuses on blood pressure control, volume management, and a search for precipitating factors, such as ischemia or dysrhythmias.

Blood pressure control
Control of underlying hypertension is the most important objective when treating HFpEF. Studies evaluating specific drug classes in HFpEF have not shown a clear superiority, and treatment may require multiple agents. Hypertension should be treated to a goal systolic blood pressure less than 130 mm Hg.[26]

Volume management

Diuretics should be used to control the symptoms of volume overload in patients with HFpEF. Similar to patients with HFrEF, the use of loop diuretics is effective. An aldosterone antagonist may be considered in patients who meet the following criteria: EF greater than 45%, elevated BNP or HF admission within 1 year, glomerular filtration rate greater than 30 mL/min, creatinine less than 2.5 mg/dL, and potassium less than 5.0 mEq/L.[26] This new recommendation is based on the Treatment of Preserved Cardiac Function Heart Failure with an Aldosterone Antagonist (TOPCAT) trial, which found that treatment with spironolactone reduced hospitalization rates in patients with HFpEF.[63]

Statins

Many patients with HFpEF have underlying CAD, so at-risk individuals should receive statin therapy according to the current guideline recommendations.

Other considerations

In patients who present with HFpEF exacerbations, investigate for underlying causes, including ischemia and atrial fibrillation. Data are lacking regarding the role of coronary revascularization in the treatment of chronic HFpEF. Revascularization is a consideration if ischemic heart disease is thought to be contributing to underlying symptoms.[3] Atrial fibrillation may worsen HF symptoms in patients with HFpEF because of the impaired filling time and deficient synchronized atrial contraction leading to lower end diastolic volumes. Patients with HFpEF and concomitant atrial fibrillation may benefit from referral to a HF specialist.

SELF-MANAGEMENT

Self-management of HF is potentially the most critical component of disease management and (when done well) a key element to preventing HF exacerbations and unnecessary hospitalizations. Many of the common causes of acute HF exacerbations are a result of breakdowns in self-management, such as medication noncompliance, dietary indiscretion, and accelerated hypertension. Although medication titration and lifestyle guidance is paramount to setting patients with HF on the right path, it is the adherence to medication plans, participation in exercise, self-monitoring, and dietary choices that are the difference makers in clinical terms.

Every effort should be made to ensure that patients with HF understand the importance of goal-directed medical therapy to improve their mortality and prevent clinical worsening of their condition. The potential barriers to adherence with prescribed medical regimens, such as cost, patient preferences and beliefs, lack of understanding of the purpose and goals of medications, and unreported side effects of medications, should be thoroughly explored.

Physical activity is one of the most beneficial management strategies in HF. Exercise improves functional capacity and overall mortality in patients with HF.[64] In addition to the direct health benefits of physical activity, it is also a helpful tool to gauge more subtle worsening in functional capacity. Both the ACC and the European Society of cardiology recommend regular exercise as safe and effective in patients with HF.

High sodium intake frequently contributes to acute HF exacerbations. A low-sodium diet (<2 g sodium per day) is typically recommended to prevent acute volume overload. Controversy exists, however, on what the appropriate exact amount of sodium is for daily intake. Some studies have shown a worsening neurohormonal profile and, in some cases, suboptimal patient outcomes with rigid sodium restriction.[65]

Although the average daily sodium intake in the United States is around 3400 mg, single entrées at commercial restaurants often exceed 3000 mg. Patients with HF should be warned about the sodium content in commercially prepared and processed foods and should aim for a daily sodium intake of less than 2.5 to 3.0 g daily to prevent exacerbations.

Fluid restriction in patients with HF is controversial and perhaps best reserved for patients with advanced disease. Historically, hospitalized patients with HF are placed on relatively strict fluid restrictions. Although this strategy makes tracking fluid intake and output easier for the clinical team, data indicate that fluid restriction has no impact on the time to clinical stability or hospital stay.[66] Further, adherence to these goals can potentially lead to symptomatic hypotension and a predisposition to heat injury. Fluid restriction may have a more significant role in patients with advanced HF and diuretic resistance or hyponatremia. No specific fluid restriction goals are recommended by the ACC/AHA's HF management guidelines.[3]

Self-monitoring strategies can help reinforce compliance with medications and exercise regimens and serve as early warning systems for HF exacerbations. Monitoring daily weights can suggest occult fluid retention and help guide changes in outpatient medical management. Patients with HF should follow daily weights and contact their health care team in the setting of rapid and unexpected weight gain, which could be a clue to an early HF exacerbation.

SUMMARY

HF is a major cause of morbidity and mortality and represents a significant burden on health care systems. Given the expected increase in HF prevalence associated with an aging population, it is imperative to implement evidence-based solutions at the individual and systems level. Primary care clinicians are well positioned to identify risk factors, document the presence of structural heart disease, and play a central role in team-based management of patients with HF.

REFERENCES

1. Ponikowski P, Voors AA, Anker SD, et al. 2016 ESC guidelines for the diagnosis and treatment of acute and chronic heart failure: the task force for the diagnosis and treatment of acute and chronic heart failure of the European Society of Cardiology (ESC) developed with the special contribution of the Heart Failure Association (HFA) of the ESC. Eur Heart J 2016;37(27):2129–200.
2. Mann DL, Zipes DP, Libby P, et al. Braunwald's heart disease: a textbook of cardiovascular medicine. 10th edition. Philadelphia: Elsevier/Saunders; 2015.
3. Yancy CW, Jessup M, Bozkurt B, et al. 2013 ACCF/AHA guideline for the management of heart failure: executive summary: a report of the American College of Cardiology Foundation/American Heart Association Task Force on practice guidelines. Circulation 2013;128(16):1810–52.
4. Loehr LR, Rosamond WD, Chang PP, et al. Heart failure incidence and survival (from the Atherosclerosis Risk in Communities study). Am J Cardiol 2008; 101(7):1016–22.
5. Writing Group Members, Mozaffarian D, Benjamin EJ, Go AS, et al. Heart disease and stroke statistics-2016 update: a report from the American Heart Association. Circulation 2016;133(4):e38–360.
6. Heidenreich PA, Albert NM, Allen LA, et al. Forecasting the impact of heart failure in the United States: a policy statement from the American Heart Association. Circ Heart Fail 2013;6(3):606–19.

7. Voigt J, Sasha John M, Taylor A, et al. A reevaluation of the costs of heart failure and its implications for allocation of health resources in the United States. Clin Cardiol 2014;37(5):312–21.

8. Dall TM. Physician workforce shortages: what do the data really say? Acad Med 2015;90(12):1581–2.

9. Aneja S, Ross JS, Wang Y, et al. US cardiologist workforce from 1995 to 2007: modest growth, lasting geographic maldistribution especially in rural areas. Health Aff (Millwood) 2011;30(12):2301–9.

10. Writing Committee Members, Yancy CW, Jessup M, Bozkurt B, et al. 2013 ACCF/AHA guideline for the management of heart failure: a report of the American College of Cardiology Foundation/American Heart Association Task Force on Practice Guidelines. Circulation 2013;128(16):e240–327.

11. Ammar KA, Jacobsen SJ, Mahoney DW, et al. Prevalence and prognostic significance of heart failure stages: application of the American College of Cardiology/American Heart Association heart failure staging criteria in the community. Circulation 2007;115(12):1563–70.

12. Mirand AL, Beehler GP, Kuo CL, et al. Explaining the de-prioritization of primary prevention: physicians' perceptions of their role in the delivery of primary care. BMC Public Health 2003;3:15.

13. He J, Ogden LG, Bazzano LA, et al. Risk factors for congestive heart failure in US men and women: NHANES I epidemiologic follow-up study. Arch Intern Med 2001;161(7):996–1002.

14. Echouffo-Tcheugui JB, Erqou S, Butler J, et al. Assessing the risk of progression from asymptomatic left ventricular dysfunction to overt heart failure: a systematic overview and meta-analysis. JACC Heart Fail 2016;4(4):237–48.

15. Thibodeau JT, Turer AT, Gualano SK, et al. Characterization of a novel symptom of advanced heart failure: bendopnea. JACC Heart Fail 2014;2(1):24–31.

16. Falk RH. "Bendopnea" or "kamptopnea?": some thoughts on terminology and mechanisms. JACC Heart Fail 2014;2(4):425.

17. Badgett RG, Lucey CR, Mulrow CD. Can the clinical examination diagnose left-sided heart failure in adults? JAMA 1997;277(21):1712–9.

18. McKee PA, Castelli WP, McNamara PM, et al. The natural history of congestive heart failure: the Framingham study. N Engl J Med 1971;285(26):1441–6.

19. Carlson KJ, Lee DC, Goroll AH, et al. An analysis of physicians' reasons for prescribing long-term digitalis therapy in outpatients. J Chronic Dis 1985;38(9):733–9.

20. Roger VL. Epidemiology of heart failure. Circ Res 2013;113(6):646–59.

21. Pinkerman C, Sander P, Breeding J, et al. Health care guideline: heart failure in adults. Institute for Clinical Systems Improvement; 2013. p. 2013.

22. Madias JE. ECG changes and voltage attenuation in congestive heart failure. Hosp Chron 2008;3(3):112–5.

23. Lin DC, Diamandis EP, Januzzi JL Jr, et al. Natriuretic peptides in heart failure. Clin Chem 2014;60(8):1040–6.

24. Beckett NS, Peters R, Fletcher AE, et al. Treatment of hypertension in patients 80 years of age or older. N Engl J Med 2008;358(18):1887–98.

25. Sciarretta S, Palano F, Tocci G, et al. Antihypertensive treatment and development of heart failure in hypertension: a Bayesian network meta-analysis of studies in patients with hypertension and high cardiovascular risk. Arch Intern Med 2011;171(5):384–94.

26. Yancy CW, Jessup M, Bozkurt B, et al. 2017 ACC/AHA/HFSA focused update of the 2013 ACCF/AHA guideline for the management of heart failure: a report of the

American College of Cardiology/American Heart Association Task Force on Clinical Practice Guidelines and the Heart Failure Society of America. Circulation 2017;136(6):e137–61.

27. American College of Cardiology Foundation Appropriate Use Criteria Task Force, American Society of Echocardiography, American Heart Association, et al. ACCF/ASE/AHA/ASNC/HFSA/HRS/SCAI/SCCM/SCCT/SCMR 2011 appropriate use criteria for echocardiography. a report of the American College of Cardiology Foundation Appropriate Use Criteria Task Force, American Society of Echocardiography, American Heart Association, American Society of Nuclear Cardiology, Heart Failure Society of America, Heart Rhythm Society, Society for Cardiovascular Angiography and Interventions, Society of Critical Care Medicine, Society of Cardiovascular Computed Tomography, Society for Cardiovascular Magnetic Resonance American College of Chest Physicians. J Am Soc Echocardiogr 2011;24(3):229–67.

28. Stone NJ, Robinson JG, Lichtenstein AH, et al. 2013 ACC/AHA guideline on the treatment of blood cholesterol to reduce atherosclerotic cardiovascular risk in adults: a report of the American College of Cardiology/American Heart Association Task Force on practice guidelines. Circulation 2014;129(25 Suppl 2):S1–45.

29. Lind M, Bounias I, Olsson M, et al. Glycaemic control and incidence of heart failure in 20,985 patients with type 1 diabetes: an observational study. Lancet 2011; 378(9786):140–6.

30. Bibbins-Domingo K, Lin F, Vittinghoff E, et al. Predictors of heart failure among women with coronary disease. Circulation 2004;110(11):1424–30.

31. Berl T, Hunsicker LG, Lewis JB, et al. Cardiovascular outcomes in the Irbesartan Diabetic Nephropathy Trial of patients with type 2 diabetes and overt nephropathy. Ann Intern Med 2003;138(7):542–9.

32. Mills EJ, Rachlis B, Wu P, et al. Primary prevention of cardiovascular mortality and events with statin treatments: a network meta-analysis involving more than 65,000 patients. J Am Coll Cardiol 2008;52(22):1769–81.

33. Braunwald E, Domanski MJ, Fowler SE, et al. Angiotensin-converting-enzyme inhibition in stable coronary artery disease. N Engl J Med 2004;351(20):2058–68.

34. Wilhelmsen L, Rosengren A, Eriksson H, et al. Heart failure in the general population of men–morbidity, risk factors and prognosis. J Intern Med 2001;249(3): 253–61.

35. Redfield MM, Jacobsen SJ, Burnett JC, et al. Burden of systolic and diastolic ventricular dysfunction in the community: appreciating the scope of the heart failure epidemic. JAMA 2003;289(2):194–202.

36. McDonagh TA, Morrison CE, Lawrence A, et al. Symptomatic and asymptomatic left-ventricular systolic dysfunction in an urban population. Lancet 1997; 350(9081):829–33.

37. Jong P, Yusuf S, Rousseau MF, et al. Effect of enalapril on 12-year survival and life expectancy in patients with left ventricular systolic dysfunction: a follow-up study. Lancet 2003;361(9372):1843–8.

38. Garg R, Yusuf S. Overview of randomized trials of angiotensin-converting enzyme inhibitors on mortality and morbidity in patients with heart failure. Collaborative Group on ACE Inhibitor Trials. JAMA 1995;273(18):1450–6.

39. Pfeffer MA, McMurray JJ, Velazquez EJ, et al. Valsartan, captopril, or both in myocardial infarction complicated by heart failure, left ventricular dysfunction, or both. N Engl J Med 2003;349(20):1893–906.

40. Effect of metoprolol CR/XL in chronic heart failure: metoprolol CR/XL randomised intervention trial in congestive heart failure (MERIT-HF). Lancet 1999;353(9169): 2001–7.
41. Packer M, Fowler MB, Roecker EB, et al. Effect of carvedilol on the morbidity of patients with severe chronic heart failure: results of the carvedilol prospective randomized cumulative survival (COPERNICUS) study. Circulation 2002; 106(17):2194–9.
42. The cardiac insufficiency bisoprolol study II (CIBIS-II): a randomised trial. Lancet 1999;353(9146):9–13.
43. ALLHAT Officers and Coordinators for the ALLHAT Collaborative Research Group. The Antihypertensive and Lipid-Lowering Treatment to Prevent Heart Attack Trial. Major outcomes in high-risk hypertensive patients randomized to angiotensin-converting enzyme inhibitor or calcium channel blocker vs diuretic: the antihypertensive and lipid-lowering treatment to prevent heart attack trial (ALLHAT). JAMA 2002;288(23):2981–97.
44. Packer M, O'Connor CM, Ghali JK, et al. Effect of amlodipine on morbidity and mortality in severe chronic heart failure. Prospective Randomized Amlodipine Survival Evaluation Study Group. N Engl J Med 1996;335(15):1107–14.
45. Moss AJ, Zareba W, Hall WJ, et al. Prophylactic implantation of a defibrillator in patients with myocardial infarction and reduced ejection fraction. N Engl J Med 2002;346(12):877–83.
46. Toh S, Reichman ME, Houstoun M, et al. Comparative risk for angioedema associated with the use of drugs that target the renin-angiotensin-aldosterone system. Arch Intern Med 2012;172(20):1582–9.
47. McMurray JJ, Packer M, Desai AS, et al. Angiotensin-neprilysin inhibition versus enalapril in heart failure. N Engl J Med 2014;371(11):993–1004.
48. Entresto [package insert]. Hanover, NJ: Novartis Pharmaceuticals Corporation; 2015. Available at: https://www.pharma.us.novartis.com/sites/www.pharma.us. novartis.com/files/entresto.pdf. Accessed April 15, 2017.
49. Poole-Wilson PA, Swedberg K, Cleland JG, et al. Comparison of carvedilol and metoprolol on clinical outcomes in patients with chronic heart failure in the Carvedilol Or Metoprolol European Trial (COMET): randomised controlled trial. Lancet 2003;362(9377):7–13.
50. Pitt B, Zannad F, Remme WJ, et al. The effect of spironolactone on morbidity and mortality in patients with severe heart failure. Randomized Aldactone Evaluation Study Investigators. N Engl J Med 1999;341(10):709–17.
51. Zannad F, McMurray JJ, Krum H, et al. Eplerenone in patients with systolic heart failure and mild symptoms. N Engl J Med 2011;364(1):11–21.
52. Taylor AL, Ziesche S, Yancy C, et al. Combination of isosorbide dinitrate and hydralazine in blacks with heart failure. N Engl J Med 2004;351(20):2049–57.
53. Hardin EA, Grodin JL. Diuretic strategies in acute decompensated heart failure. Curr Heart Fail Rep 2017;14(2):127–33.
54. Fox K, Ford I, Steg PG, et al, BEAUTIFUL Investigators. Ivabradine for patients with stable coronary artery disease and left-ventricular systolic dysfunction (BEAUTIFUL): a randomised, double-blind, placebo-controlled trial. Lancet 2008;372(9641):807–16.
55. Swedberg K, Komajda M, Böhm M, et al. Ivabradine and outcomes in chronic heart failure (SHIFT): a randomised placebo-controlled study. Lancet 2010; 376(9744):875–85.
56. Digitalis Investigation Group. The effect of digoxin on mortality and morbidity in patients with heart failure. N Engl J Med 1997;336(8):525–33.

57. Bardy GH, Lee KL, Mark DB, et al. Amiodarone or an implantable cardioverter-defibrillator for congestive heart failure. N Engl J Med 2005;352(3):225–37.
58. Rose EA, Gelijns AC, Moskowitz AJ, et al. Long-term use of a left ventricular assist device for end-stage heart failure. N Engl J Med 2001;345(20):1435–43.
59. Bagchi AD, Esposito D, Kim M, et al. Utilization of, and adherence to, drug therapy among Medicaid beneficiaries with congestive heart failure. Clin Ther 2007; 29(8):1771–83.
60. Neily JB, Toto KH, Gardner EB, et al. Potential contributing factors to noncompliance with dietary sodium restriction in patients with heart failure. Am Heart J 2002;143(1):29–33.
61. Braun LT, Grady KL, Kutner JS, et al. Palliative care and cardiovascular disease and stroke: a policy statement from the American Heart Association/American Stroke Association. Circulation 2016;134(11):e198–225.
62. Allen LA, Stevenson LW, Grady KL, et al. Decision making in advanced heart failure: a scientific statement from the American Heart Association. Circulation 2012; 125(15):1928–52.
63. Pitt B, Pfeffer MA, Assmann SF, et al. Spironolactone for heart failure with preserved ejection fraction. N Engl J Med 2014;370(15):1383–92.
64. Piepoli MF, Davos C, Francis DP, et al. Exercise training meta-analysis of trials in patients with chronic heart failure (ExTraMATCH). BMJ 2004;328(7433):189.
65. Paterna S, Gaspare P, Fasullo S, et al. Normal-sodium diet compared with low-sodium diet in compensated congestive heart failure: is sodium an old enemy or a new friend? Clin Sci (Lond) 2008;114(3):221–30.
66. Travers B, O'Loughlin C, Murphy NF, et al. Fluid restriction in the management of decompensated heart failure: no impact on time to clinical stability. J Card Fail 2007;13(2):128–32.

Valvular Heart Disease

Zorana Mrsic, MD[a], Scott P. Hopkins, MD[a], Jared L. Antevil, MD[b],
Philip S. Mullenix, MD[b],*

KEYWORDS

- Valvular heart disease • Aortic stenosis • Aortic regurgitation • Mitral stenosis
- Mitral regurgitation

KEY POINTS

- Valvular heart disease can be categorized as congenital or acquired, and primary or secondary. The surveillance and recommendations for intervention and management are based on these differences.
- Basic understanding of pathologic murmurs is important for appropriate referral from primary care.
- Echocardiography is the gold standard for the diagnosis and grading of severity of valvular heart disease.
- All patients with progressive valvular heart disease should be followed annually by cardiology and surveillance imaging should be performed based on the severity of valvular dysfunction.
- In most cases, surgery or intervention is recommended only when symptoms dictate or when changes in left ventricular function have occurred. Surgery or intervention should only be performed after being discussed by a heart team that includes both cardiologists and cardiac surgeons.

INTRODUCTION

The intent of this article is to outline the diagnosis and management of commonly occurring valvular heart diseases for the office-based primary care provider in general clinical practice. The key concepts include (1) the understanding that valvular heart disease is generally categorized as either congenital or acquired, and can present in either primary or secondary fashion. Furthermore, (2) the surveillance programs, management strategies, and recommendations for intervention are based on these differences. Importantly, (3) a basic understanding of pathologic murmurs is important for appropriate referral from primary care and (4) echocardiography is the gold standard

Disclosure Statement: None
[a] Department of Medicine, Division of Cardiology, Walter Reed National Military Medical Center, 8901 Rockville Pike, Bethesda, MD 20889, USA; [b] Department of Surgery, Division of and Cardiothoracic Surgery, Walter Reed National Military Medical Center, 8901 Rockville Pike, Bethesda, MD 20889, USA
* Corresponding author.
E-mail address: philip.s.mullenix.mil@mail.mil

for the diagnosis and grading of severity of valvular heart disease. All patients with progressive valvular heart disease should (5) be followed annually by cardiology and (6) surveillance imaging should be performed based on the severity of valvular dysfunction. In most cases, (7) surgery or intervention is recommended only when symptoms dictate or when changes in left ventricular (LV) function have occurred. Finally, (8) it is important to emphasize that surgery or intervention should only be performed after being discussed by a multidisciplinary heart team that includes both cardiologists and cardiac surgeons.

ANATOMY AND PATHOPHYSIOLOGY

The heart has 4 valves that promote circulation through the heart, pulmonary, and systemic circulation. The atrioventricular valves (mitral and tricuspid) separate the atria and the ventricles. These valves are open during diastole, allowing the ventricles to fill. The semilunar valves (aortic and pulmonic) are open during systole as blood travels from the heart to the systemic and pulmonary circulations. Valvular pathologic conditions lead to either stenosis or regurgitation. Stenotic valves restrict flow. Regurgitant valves allow blood to flow back across the closed valve into the preceding chamber. The aortic valve has no regurgitation in its physiologic state, whereas the other 3 valves have elements of physiologic regurgitation. Valvular pathologic conditions are further categorized into acquired or congenital. In general, the heart can withstand significant amounts of stenosis and regurgitation before clinical symptoms appear. These symptoms are unique to each valvular pathologic condition. The end stage of most valvular heart disease is heart failure. The goals of treatment are to maintain adequate hemodynamics (blood pressure and heart rate control), manage existing arrhythmias, and treat or prevent concomitant cardiac disease (coronary heart disease, arrhythmias, and stroke).

Symptoms and signs of valvular heart disease provide important clues about the origin of specific valvular lesions. Transthoracic echocardiography (TTE) is used to diagnose and grade valvular lesions. If TTE is inadequate, other noninvasive and invasive techniques (MRI, transesophageal echocardiogram, heart catheterization) are available to characterize valvular disease. TTE is also used to monitor the progression of valvular disease. Valvular interventions are considered after the onset of symptoms but before irreversible cardiomyopathy has developed. In some cases, intervention is indicated in the absence of symptoms when there is early evidence of valve-related decline in cardiac function. This article describes the most common adult pathologic valvular diseases, as well as some of the transcatheter and surgical options available to replace or repair valves. Although surgery has long been standard practice, recent developments in transcatheter techniques are reshaping the clinical approach to patients with severe valvular heart disease.

AORTIC STENOSIS
Etiologic Factors

Aortic stenosis (AS) is primarily caused by congenital malformations of the valve, calcification of normal trileaflet valve, and rheumatic disease. Congenital aortic valve malformations include unicuspid and bicuspid valves. The bicuspid form is more common.[1] Unicuspid valves typically produce severe symptoms in infancy. Bicuspid valves present with symptomatic stenosis later in life and when superimposed calcific changes result in clinically significant valvular obstruction. Congenital lesions of the aortic valve are commonly inherited in an autosomal dominant pattern.[2]

Calcific aortic valve disease, or degenerative valve disease, is the most common cause of AS in adults.[3] It is thought to be caused by proliferative and inflammatory changes that lead to calcium deposition and an associated reduction in the mobility of the valve cusps. Rheumatic AS is caused by adhesions and fusion of the commissures and cusps, resulting in reduction in the size of the valve orifice. With reduction in the incidence of rheumatic fever in developed countries, the incidence of rheumatic heart disease has declined.[4] Rheumatic heart disease remains a problem in developing countries.

Pathophysiology

Changes to valvular form precede changes in valvular function. Changes in valve structure lead to outflow obstruction. Once this occurs, progression is inevitable. The rate of progression from mild to severe outflow obstruction is variable, taking anywhere from several years to more than a decade. Although the degree of stenosis required to produce symptoms varies between patients, clinically significant AS is associated with severe outflow obstruction. Chronic obstruction of the LV outflow tract leads to LV pressure overload. This results in LV hypertrophy, diastolic dysfunction, increased oxygen consumption, ischemia, and LV systolic dysfunction.

Symptoms

Symptoms of AS include decreased exercise tolerance, fatigue, dyspnea, angina, syncope. Symptoms typically manifest at around age 50 to 70 years in patients with bicuspid aortic valve stenosis, and after the age of 70 in patients with calcific AS.[5] Angina can occur in patients with severe AS regardless of the degree of coronary artery occlusion. In patients without significant coronary artery disease, angina is caused by increased myocardial oxygen demand of the hypertrophied myocardium, and the reduced oxygen delivery secondary to shortened diastole and compression of coronary arteries by the stenotic valvular annulus. Syncope is caused by an exercise-induced drop in systemic blood pressure in the setting of fixed cardiac output, leading to cerebral hypoperfusion. These symptoms, as well as symptoms of heart failure, indicate stages of AS. Aortic valve interventions are typically performed before the development of heart failure symptoms.

Murmur

The murmur of AS is classically a late-peaking systolic murmur, radiating to the carotid arteries bilaterally and best heard in the aortic area. The murmur may contain a high-frequency component radiating to the apex that can be mistaken for a murmur of mitral regurgitation (MR; Gallavardin phenomenon).[6] The intensity of the AS murmur does not correlate directly with the severity of AS. As the LV fails and stroke volume decreases, the murmur becomes softer and can disappear entirely. The timing of the peak of the murmur, however, does correlate with the severity of the AS. Later-peaking murmurs correlate with more severe AS.

In addition to classic auscultatory findings, severe AS is also manifested by abnormal carotid upstroke and cardiac impulse. The carotid upstroke is a slow rising, low-amplitude pulse with a late peak known as pulsus parvus et tardus. This finding is specific for severe AS; its absence, however, does not rule out severe valve stenosis. The cardiac impulse in severe AS is typically sustained. As patients develop progressive LV failure, the impulse displaces inferiorly and laterally. With severe AS, the systolic blood pressure and pulse pressure may be reduced. Neither of these findings, however, are sensitive or specific.

Diagnosis

Echocardiography is the standard modality for the diagnosis and surveillance of AS.[7,8] Echocardiography allows for visualization of valve anatomy, assessment of the severity of valvular calcification, and calculation of hemodynamic parameters surrounding the valvular orifice. Echocardiography can allow measurement of the transaortic jet velocity and calculation of the mean transaortic pressure gradient and the area of the valvular orifice. Severe AS is defined by an aortic jet velocity greater than or equal to 4 m/s or a mean pressure gradient greater than or equal to 40 mm Hg in the presence of normal cardiac output. Severe AS is also characterized by an effective aortic valve area less than or equal to 1 cm^2 or less than 0.6 cm^2/m^2. In addition to valve assessment, echocardiography allows assessment of LV function. In the presence of severe AS, a significant decline in cardiac function indicates the need for intervention irrespective of the presence or absence of associated symptoms. If echocardiography does not provide adequate evaluation of valve anatomy or hemodynamics, cardiac magnetic resonance (CMR) is an acceptable alternative. Computed tomography can be used to evaluate aortic anatomy, which helps in planning for valve intervention procedures.[9] Combined with the history and physical examination, noninvasive testing is typically sufficient to diagnose severe AS. If noninvasive testing is inconclusive, cardiac catheterization and direct measurement of the transaortic pressure gradient can be performed. Coronary angiography is often performed in patients with concomitant coronary artery disease risk factors to evaluate coronary artery stenosis before a planned single procedure.

Surveillance and Referral

AS is a progressive disease with heterogeneity in rates of progression between patients. Because it is impossible to predict rates of progression for individual patients, close clinical and echocardiographic follow-up is indicated for all patients with asymptomatic AS, even in mild to moderate stages.[7,8] For patients with mild AS and an aortic jet velocity 2.0 to 2.9 m/s, repeat evaluation should be performed every 3 to 5 years. Patients with moderate AS, and an aortic jet velocity 3.0 to 3.9 m/s, should be evaluated every 1 to 2 years. With severe AS (aortic jet velocity $\geq$4 m/s), the rate of progression to symptoms is high and repeat evaluation should occur every 6 months to 1 year. If the symptom status is unclear, physician-monitored exercise testing can help uncover clinically relevant symptoms and hemodynamic changes (eg, decrease in systolic blood pressure). Exercise testing should be avoided in symptomatic patients. In patients with known AS, a change in physical examination with increase in murmur intensity or development of relevant clinical symptoms should prompt a repeat TTE. Patients with asymptomatic, mild to moderate AS can be followed in the primary care setting with serial clinical evaluation and echocardiography. Patients with symptomatic moderate AS or severe AS (whether symptomatic or not) should be followed by a cardiologist.

Indications for Intervention

The current American College of Cardiology/American Heart Association Task Force (ACC/AHA) indications for surgical or interventional cardiology intervention for AS with either aortic valve replacement (AVR) or transcatheter AVR (TAVR) include (1) symptomatic patients with severe high-gradients, (2) asymptomatic patients with severe disease and LV ejection fraction (LVEF) less than 50%, and (3) patients with severe (in select cases, moderate) disease undergoing other cardiac surgery.[7,10] Intervention is also reasonable for (1) low-risk asymptomatic patients with very severe

AS (aortic velocity $\geq$5 m/s); (2) those with severe asymptomatic disease but with decreased exercise tolerance or an decline in blood pressure due to exercise; and (3) symptomatic patients with low-flow or low-gradient severe AS and a low-dose dobutamine stress study with aortic velocity greater than or equal to 4.0 m/s and a valve area less than or equal to 1.0 cm^2, or who are normotensive with LVEF greater than or equal to 50% and valve obstruction is most likely cause of symptoms. Currently, surgical AVR is generally offered to low-risk and intermediate-risk patients, and TAVR to high-risk or prohibitive-risk surgical patients, although these data comparing surgical and transcatheter approaches to AVR are in evolution and continuing to mature.

AORTIC REGURGITATION
Etiologic Factors

Aortic regurgitation (AR) is caused by disease of the aortic valve leaflets or the wall of the aortic root. AR due to dilation of the ascending aorta is more common than primary valvular disease.[11] Numerous conditions lead to aortic root dilation, including age-related degeneration, cystic medial necrosis (with or without Marfan syndrome), dilation associated with bicuspid aortic valves, syphilitic aortitis, seronegative spondyloarthropathies, giant cell arteritis, hypertension, and aortic dissection. There are also several primary valvular causes of AR. Infective endocarditis is among the more common causes of acute AR and it can be caused by either vegetation that prevents leaflet coaptation or valve leaflet perforation. In addition to developing stenosis, bicuspid aortic valves can also become regurgitant over time due to incomplete valve closure and/or leaflet prolapse. In this setting, degeneration and calcification of aortic valves lead to mixed valvular stenosis and regurgitation. Less common causes of AR include autoimmune or connective tissues disease, vasculitides, and inflammatory bowel disease.

Pathophysiology

Aortic valve regurgitation leads to LV volume overload, increased stroke volume, and increased aortic systolic pressure, contributing to chamber hypertrophy and dilation. This leads to increased myocardial oxygen consumption. An associated decrease in effective stroke volume with a decreased diastolic time and diastolic pressure cause decreased myocardial oxygen supply. The mismatch in myocardial oxygen supply and demand leads to ischemia and LV failure.

Symptoms

Acute AR leads to an abrupt onset of symptoms, including dyspnea and chest pain. Chronic AR, however, is often initially asymptomatic due to the gradual nature of the resultant LV enlargement. Symptoms develop after the left ventricle is no longer able to compensate. Symptoms of AR are those of heart failure and include exertional dyspnea, orthopnea, and paroxysmal nocturnal dyspnea. Patients can also develop angina late in the course of the disease, which is often worse at night. This is due to a decrease coronary perfusion pressure as the result of a decreasing heart rate. This relative bradycardia prolongs diastole, leading to increased regurgitation and a decrease in arterial diastolic pressure with resultant myocardial ischemia.

Murmur

The murmur of AR is typically a high-frequency diastolic decrescendo murmur beginning immediately after the second sound (S2) of the aorta. The murmur is best heard with the diaphragm of the stethoscope, and can be accentuated by asking the patient to sit and lean forward and hold their breath at the end of expiration. The duration of the murmur correlates more with the severity of AR than the intensity. Murmurs lasting longer into diastole are associated with more severe valvular regurgitation. A middiastolic and late diastolic apical rumble is also common in severe AR. This phenomenon (Austin Flint murmur), is caused by the regurgitant jet impinging on the anterior leaflet of the mitral valve. Patients with chronic AR can also have a harsh systolic outflow murmur due to increased LV stroke volume and ejection rate.

Patients with chronic severe AR can present with a series of other interesting physical examination findings. Systolic pulsations of the uvula (Müller sign) or a systolic head bob (De Musset sign) are associated with AR.[12] Patients often have a prominent arterial pulse, with an abrupt distention and quick collapse (water hammer or Corrigan pulse). A bisferiens (double peak) pulse can sometimes be palpated. The apical impulse is diffuse and hyperdynamic and often displaced inferiorly and laterally. Arterial systolic pressure is often elevated with a low diastolic pressure, leading to a widened pulse pressure.

Diagnosis

Echocardiography is also the primary modality for diagnosing and following AR.[7,8] It allows visualization of the valve anatomy, the ascending aorta, and the LV size and function, and helps quantify the degree of valve regurgitation. In severe AR, the central jet width (as assessed by color flow Doppler) is greater than 65% of the LV outflow track, the regurgitant volume greater than or equal to 60 mL per beat, and the regurgitant fraction greater than or equal to 50%. If echocardiography is suboptimal, cardiac MRI can provide structural information and a more accurate evaluation of regurgitant volumes and LV size and function.[13] If CMR is unavailable or contraindicated, cardiac catheterization can performed.

Surveillance or Referral

Patients with known AR should be followed routinely for clinical symptoms and signs of heart failure.[7,8] Patients with mild AR should undergo TTE every 3 to 5 years, whereas those with moderate AR should undergo TTE every 1 to 2 years. Once patients develop severe AR, TTE screening should be every 6 to 12 months.

Indications for Intervention

The current ACC/AHA indications for surgical intervention for AR with AVR include (1) symptomatic patients with severe AR regardless of systolic function, (2) asymptomatic patients with severe disease and LVEF less than 50%, and (3) patients with severe (in select cases, moderate) disease undergoing other cardiac surgery.[7,10] Intervention is also reasonable for (1) asymptomatic patients with severe (in some cases, moderate) disease who are undergoing cardiac surgery for other indications and (2) asymptomatic patients with severe disease and normal LVEF but with severe LV dilation (>50 mm LVESD or >65 mm LVEDD) if surgical risk is low.

MITRAL STENOSIS

Rheumatic heart disease remains the most common cause of mitral stenosis (MS) worldwide.[4] Although less common in developed countries, rheumatic heart disease is still a significant problem in the developing world. In patients with rheumatic heart disease, 25% will have isolated MS and 40% will have combined MS and MR. The progression of disease is variable and likely depends on recurrence of rheumatic fever. It is not unusual for it to take up to 20 years for MS to develop. Rheumatic MS is characterized by thickened leaflet tips, fusion of the mitral commissures, and chordal shortening. Early in the disease process, the valve remains flexible and snaps open. Subsequent restriction of valvular leaflets that do not fully open causes a classic doming appearance. With commissural fusion, a small central (fish-mouth) orifice develops.

Other causes of MS include cardiac tumors, endocarditis, and mitral annular calcification. These causes mimic rheumatic MS hemodynamically and have a similar clinical presentation. These disorders are not, however, treated the same way as rheumatic MS and should not be considered true valvular stenosis. Mitral annular calcification is common in patients with calcific AS. The stenosis of mitral annular calcification is sometimes referred to as functional MS, and rarely causes a severe inflow gradient. There is no specific treatment of mitral annular calcification. When present and severe, however, it carries a poor prognosis.

Pathophysiology

The degree of MS is defined by the mitral orifice area.[14] The normal orifice is 4 to 6 cm^2. Mild MS is less than or equal to 2 cm^2, severe is less than or equal to 1.5 cm^2, and very severe is less than or equal to 1 cm^2. As the orifice area decreases, a higher left atrial pressure is required to maintain LV filling and cardiac output. As left atrial pressures increase, there is an increase in pulmonary venous pressure leading to dyspnea. The left ventricle is physiologically normal in MS though it may be small and underfilled. The filling of the left ventricle depends on both the left atrial pressure and the diastolic filling time. With tachycardia (during exercise or with an atrial arrhythmia), diastolic filling time shortens, leading to worsening symptoms. In normal sinus rhythm, as the left atrium contracts there is a kick that provides additional ventricular filling. When this filling contribution is diminished (eg, atrial fibrillation or significant tachycardia), symptoms of dyspnea worsen. Underfilling of the left ventricle (with an associated decrease in cardiac output) exacerbates other symptoms of heart failure such as fatigue and exercise intolerance. Other hemodynamic consequences include increased pulmonary arterial pressure and symptoms of right heart failure. With stasis in the left atrium, the risk of thrombus formation and systemic embolism can increase significantly as well.

Symptoms

Symptoms of MS are often insidious in onset. Classic symptoms include fatigue, dyspnea, and decreased exercise tolerance. Patients often attribute the latter to deconditioning and may change their lifestyle to compensate for the lack of exercise tolerance. Other (less common) symptoms include hemoptysis, isolated chest pain (usually due to severe pulmonary edema), and hoarseness (compression of the recurrent laryngeal nerve by the left atrium).

Physical Examination and Diagnosis

Physical examination findings in patients with chronic severe MS are most often attributable to atrial fibrillation and heart failure. Mitral facies (pink-purple patches on the face) are occasionally present and thought to be due to systemic vasoconstriction. Auscultation reveals an opening snap (OS) and loud first sound (S1) if the valve is still flexible enough. With worsening pulmonary hypertension, a split S2 develops. The murmur occurs during diastole and is low-pitched. It is best heard in the left lateral recumbent position with the bell of the stethoscope. The length of the murmur correlates with the severity of the stenosis.

Echocardiography is the primary modality for diagnosing and grading the severity of MS.[7,8] Echocardiographic findings include thickening, restriction, and doming of the mitral leaflets. There is often commissural fusion, thickening, and calcification. The chorda tendinae tend to be thickened as well. Calculated valve area and mean transmitral pressure gradient help grade the severity. Other standard echocardiographic measurements include left atrial size, pulmonary arterial pressure, left or right ventricular size and function, and assessment of the other valves for evidence of rheumatic changes. A simple scoring technique compiles these echocardiographic findings to determine whether the valve is amenable to percutaneous balloon valvotomy. Transesophageal echocardiography is only necessary if there is poor image quality or a need for valve planimetry. Stress echocardiography can be used to assess exercise tolerance and exertional pulmonary pressures. ECG findings associated with MS can include left atrial enlargement, atrial fibrillation, and right ventricular hypertrophy. Chest radiograph findings often show left atrial enlargement and evidence of pulmonary congestion. Left heart catheterization is used to measure the transmitral gradient and calculate the valve area, most often during percutaneous valvotomy. The natural history of severe MR without surgical correction is a 5-year survival of 60% in patients with New York Heart Association (NYHA) III symptoms and 15% in patients with NYHA IV symptoms.[15]

Surveillance and Referral

All patients with MS should be evaluated with history and examination annually.[7,8] Echocardiography should be performed every 3 to 5 years for mild MS, every 1 to 2 years for moderate MS, and annually for severe MS. Patients with evidence of rheumatic heart disease should be treated with appropriate antibiotic prophylaxis.[16] Other treatments target complications of MS, including heart failure, atrial fibrillation, and the prevention of thromboembolic disease.

Indications for Intervention

The current ACC/AHA indications for intervention for MS outline that percutaneous mitral valve balloon commissurotomy (PMBC) may be considered for symptomatic patients with severe MS ($\leq$1.5 cm^2) and favorable valve morphology in the absence of contraindications.[7,10] Surgical mitral valve replacement is indicated in (1) patients with severe MS who are not high risk for surgery and are not candidates for or failed previous PMBC and (2) patients with severe MS undergoing other cardiac surgery. PMBC is reasonable for asymptomatic patients with very severe MS and favorable valve morphology in the absence of contraindications, and can be considered in high or prohibitive surgical risk patients. Mitral valve surgery is reasonable for severely symptomatic patients with severe MS provided there are other operative indications. It can be considered in select other situations, including hemodynamically significant MS during exercise, or recurrent embolic events while receiving adequate anticoagulation if mitral valve replacement is combined with excision of the left atrial appendage.

MITRAL REGURGITATION

The mitral valve apparatus is composed of an annulus, 2 leaflets, chordae tendinae, and papillary muscles. The surrounding left ventricle also contributes the shape and the function of the mitral valve. Defects in any of these components can result in MR. Recent classification schemes divide MR into primary and secondary causes.[17] Primary MR is caused by defects in the mitral leaflets, chordae, and papillary muscles. This includes mitral valve prolapse (MVP), rheumatic MR, infective endocarditis, and penetrating trauma. Secondary MR is caused by changes to the shape or function of the left ventricle or mitral annulus. Common causes of secondary MR are ischemia, hypertrophic cardiomyopathy, and mitral annular calcification. The identification of primary or secondary MR is important because the indication for and outcomes of surgical repair or replacement vary significantly.

The most common cause of primary MR is MVP. It is estimated that approximately 3% of the population has some degree of prolapse of the mitral valve.[18] MVP is more common in women who also tend to have examination findings at a younger age and a more benign course than men. The clinical findings associated with MVP include a systolic click and midsystolic to late systolic murmur. The echocardiographic findings include displacement of 1 or both of the leaflets 2 mm beyond the annular plane in the long axis view. MVP is generally a primary condition but can also be seen with hereditary connective tissue disorders, including Marfan syndrome and Ehlers-Danlos syndrome.

Pathophysiology

In acute MR, the LV afterload decreases significantly and the ventricle does not have adequate time to dilate, resulting in a reduced end diastolic ventricular volume. To increase the ejection fraction, the heart compensates by increasing contractility and decreasing the end systolic volume to maintain cardiac output. If the regurgitation persists, the left ventricle dilates through the process of eccentric hypertrophy, allowing the end diastolic volume to increase. The ejection fraction normalizes and cardiac output is maintained by the increase in end diastolic volume. As the dilation becomes too great, the ejection fraction decreases, cardiac output decreases, and the patient clinically decompensates. Severe MR increases left atrial pressures and pulmonary venous pressures to a lesser extent than MS. Left atrial dilation often results in atrial arrhythmias, most commonly atrial fibrillation.[19]

Symptoms

The symptoms associated with MR develop based on the rate of progression of valvular disease. This varies widely depending on the underlying causes. Dyspnea develops secondary to pulmonary congestion. Fatigue and exercise intolerance are often the result of a reduced cardiac output or atrial arrhythmias. Systemic embolization is less common than with MS.

Physical Examination and Diagnosis

Auscultation of MR reveals a diminished S1 and wide splitting of the S2 due to early aortic valve closure. The murmur is high-pitched and holosystolic. If there is associated MVP, a midsystolic to late systolic murmur and midsystolic click may be audible. An early systolic murmur may be detected in acute secondary MR. TTE is used to confirm the diagnosis and grade the severity of MR.[7,8] Echocardiographic findings consistent with severe MR include left atrial enlargement and increased systolic motion of the left ventricle. Color Doppler helps quantify the severity of MR based on the valvular orifice and transvalvular flow. Transesophageal echocardiography can further define valvular anatomy to assess for the suitability of possible repair. Cardiac MRI gives a more accurate assessment of regurgitant fraction and volume. LV angiography can qualitatively assess MR by visualizing the amount of contrast refluxing into the left atrium. LV volumes and forward stroke volume are calculated angiographically using either the Fick or thermodilution method.[20] ECG findings include left atrial enlargement and atrial arrhythmias. Chest radiograph shows cardiac enlargement and left atrial enlargement.

Surveillance and Referral

The natural history of primary MR is highly variable. Asymptomatic severe MR progresses to a symptomatic state in 30% to 40% of patients in roughly 5 years. The 5-year survival for patients with severe symptomatic MR who decline surgery is 30%.[21] The utility of medical therapy in managing MR is uncertain. Adequate control of hypertension is recommended. In acute severe MR afterload reduction improves hemodynamics and may be used to temporize a patient's condition before surgery.[22] The benefits of vasodilators are less certain in the treatment of chronic MR. Antibiotic and prophylaxis for all patients with MR is no longer recommended. Patients with severe MR and atrial fibrillation should be anticoagulated.[23]

As previously noted, MR is categorized as primary or secondary, and as mild, moderate, or severe. The 2014 ACC/AHA guidelines for the management of patients with valvular heart disease[7] define patients as at risk, progressive mild, progressive moderate, and severe. Mild MR with no evidence of progressive disease (ie, prolapse or annular dilation) does not require surveillance. Patients with progressive mild disease should have an echocardiogram every 3 to 5 years. Patients with progressive moderate MR should have an echocardiogram every 1 to 2 years. Patients with severe MR who are asymptomatic should be imaged more frequently.

Indications for Intervention

The decision to refer for surgery depends on cause, severity, and symptoms.[7,10] Unlike MS, for which surgical intervention almost always requires valve replacement, the mitral valve can often be surgically repaired in patients with MR. According to the ACC/AHA guidelines, surgical or interventional cardiology intervention for MR is recommended for (1) symptomatic patients with primary severe MR and LVEF greater than 30%, (2) asymptomatic patients with LVEF 30% to 60% and/or ventricular dilation greater than or equal to 40 mm, and (3) patients with severe (and select moderate) disease undergoing cardiac surgery for other indications. Surgical intervention is also reasonable in (1) asymptomatic patients with MR and preserved LV function without ventricular dilation in whom the likelihood of repair over replacement is greater than 95% and the expected mortality risk is less than 1%, when performed at a Heart Valve Center of Excellence and (2) those with severe MR and progressive increase in LV size or decreased LVEF even before they reach thresholds of either an LVEF less than 60% or endsystolic ventricular diameter greater than or equal to 40. Other situations that warrant consideration for surgical intervention include patients with severe MR and (1) new onset atrial fibrillation, (2) resting pulmonary hypertension, (3) in whom long-term anticoagulation is contraindicated or has questionable reliability, and (4) patients with severely depressed LVEF less than 30% with appropriate surgical risk.

TRICUSPID STENOSIS

Isolated tricuspid stenosis (TS) is uncommon. Rheumatic disease is also the most common cause for TS, which is often accompanied by AS and MS. Other rare causes of TS include tricuspid atresia, right atrial tumors, and carcinoid syndrome. A diastolic pressure gradient between the right atrium and the right ventricle defines TS. The gradient increases with inspiration and exercise, and even low gradients can elevate right atrial pressure, leading to systemic venous congestion. Severe TS[7] is defined by a mean pressure gradient greater than 5 mm Hg, pressure half-time greater than or equal to 190 milliseconds, and valve area less than or equal to 1.0 cm^2 with associated right atrial and inferior vena cava enlargement. With TS, cardiac output at rest is decreased and fails to increase with exercise. Patients typically present with fatigue.

Anasarca, ascites, hepatomegaly, dyspnea, and pulmonary edema are other presenting signs and symptoms.

Physical Examination

On auscultation, the OS of the tricuspid valve can be difficult to distinguish from a mitral OS. The tricuspid OS usually follows the mitral OS and is best heard at the left lower sternal border (the mitral OS is most prominent at the apex). The diastolic murmur of TS shares many qualities with the murmur of MS but is best heard along the left lower sternal border. Both the OS and the murmur of TS increase with inspiration, leg raises, and squatting. There is typically jugular venous distention and (for patients in sinus rhythm), large venous a wave and prominent presystolic pulsations (if the liver is enlarged) are observed.

Diagnosis

As with other valvulopathies, echocardiography is used to diagnose and assess severity of TS.[7,8] Doppler and 3-dimensional echocardiography typically provide all necessary hemodynamic and anatomic information needed for the evaluation and management of TS. If the severity of TS is unclear, cardiac catheterization with simultaneous pressure recordings in the right atrium and the right ventricle can be performed.

Management

Patients with TS are typically managed with salt restriction and diuresis.[7] In the absence of TR, patients with severe symptomatic TS can undergo percutaneous balloon commissurotomy. Because most patients have concomitant valvular regurgitation, tricuspid valve surgery is more commonly pursued for that indication.

Indications for Intervention

The AHC/ACC recommends tricuspid valve surgery for patients with (1) severe TS at the time of operation for left-sided valve disease and (2) for patients with isolated, symptomatic severe TS.[7,10]

TRICUSPID REGURGITATION

Tricuspid regurgitation (TR) often occurs secondary to left-sided valvular disease, which increases right-sided cardiac volume and pressure. The most common cause of TR is dilation of the right ventricle and the tricuspid annulus, causing poor coaptation of valve leaflets. This may occur due to LV dysfunction, in the setting of an RV infarct, or secondary to pulmonary hypertension (typically when pulmonary artery systolic pressures exceed 55 mm Hg). Primary TR occurs through processes directly affecting the tricuspid valve apparatus, including tricuspid valve prolapse, Ebstein anomaly, rheumatic heart disease, trauma, infective endocarditis, carcinoid syndrome, and cardiac tumors.

In the absence of pulmonary hypertension, TR is well-tolerated by most patients. If patients have pulmonary hypertension and TR, cardiac output declines and symptoms of right-sided heart failure develop. In this setting, patients present with weakness, fatigue, jugular venous distention, congestive hepatopathy, ascites, and peripheral edema. On examination, the patients have a prominent jugular venous systolic wave (C-V wave). A venous thrill and a murmur in the neck may be present, as well as a pulsatile liver.

On auscultation, patients may have a systolic murmur, which has different qualities depending on the presence or absence of pulmonary hypertension. In patients with pulmonary hypertension, the murmur is high pitched and pansystolic. In the absence of pulmonary hypertension, the murmur has a low intensity and is limited to the first half of systole. In both cases, the murmur increases with inspiration, exercise, and leg elevation. If tricuspid valve prolapse is present, a nonejection systolic click and a late systolic murmur can be heard along the left lower sternal border.

Diagnosis

Echocardiography is used to evaluate the tricuspid valve anatomy and degree of regurgitation.[7,8] Right ventricular size, systolic function, and estimation of pulmonary arterial pressures are routinely included. In patients with suboptimal echocardiographic windows, cardiac MRI better evaluates right ventricular size and function, leaflet anatomy, and the degree of tricuspid annular dilation. If clinical and imaging data are discordant, cardiac catheterization can be performed. Patients with severe primary TR have evidence of leaflet flail or distortion. In patients with severe functional TR, there is dilation of the tricuspid annulus to greater than 40 mm. The central jet area greater than 10 cm^2, vena contracta width greater than 0.7 cm, and systolic flow reversal of the hepatic veins also indicate severe TR.

Management

Patients without coexisting pulmonary hypertension usually tolerate regurgitation through the tricuspid valve reasonably well. When signs or symptoms of right sided heart failure develop, diuretics are first-line agents for symptom management.[7]

Indications for Intervention

The ACC/AHA guidelines outline that surgical intervention is recommended at the time of left-sided valve surgery for patients with severe TR.[7,10] Surgery can also be beneficial in patients (1) at time of left-sided valve surgery who manifest mild or moderate TR and associated tricuspid annulus dilation or pulmonary hypertension,[7] and (2) symptomatic patients with isolated severe TR unresponsive to medical therapy. Other considerations for intervention include patients with asymptomatic severe TR with associated progressive right ventricular dysfunction. Tricuspid valve repair, rather than replacement, may be possible depending on the cause and severity of TR, and is generally preferred if possible.

PULMONIC VALVE DISEASE

Most cases of pulmonic stenosis are congenital in origin. Other causes include rheumatic, carcinoid, and cardiac tumor obstruction, and external compression by a dilated aorta. Congenital pulmonic stenosis is managed by balloon dilation.[7,8] Pulmonic regurgitation (PR) is usually caused by dilation of the annulus secondary to pulmonary hypertension or dilation of the pulmonary artery. Infective endocarditis can also cause PR. An increasingly common cause of PR occurs in adults with congenital disease, such as tetralogy of Fallot, that was previously surgically corrected. Significant PR is usually tolerated very well in isolation. Treatment of PR is usually aimed at treating the cause of the pulmonary hypertension, right heart failure, or volume overload. Surgery or percutaneous approaches are used for patients with previously corrected congenital disease.

REFERENCES

1. Ward C. Clinical significance of the bicuspid aortic valve. Heart 2000;83:81–5.
2. Cripe L, Andelfinger G, Martin LJ, et al. Bicuspid aortic valve is heritable. J Am Coll Cardiol 2004;44(1):138–43.
3. Fedak PWM, Verma S, David TE, et al. Clinical and pathophysiological implications of a bicuspid aortic valve. Circulation 2002;106:900–4.
4. Seckeler MD, Hoke TR. The worldwide epidemiology of acute rheumatic fever and rheumatic heart disease. Clin Epidemiol 2011;3:67–84.
5. Pellikka PA, Sarano ME, Nishimura RA, et al. Outcome of 622 adults with asymptomatic, hemodynamically significant aortic stenosis during prolonged followup. Circulation 2005;111:3290–5.
6. Giles TD, Martinez EC, Burch GE. Gallavardin phenomenon in aortic stenosis: a possible mechanism. Arch Intern Med 1974;134(4):747–9.
7. Nishimura RA, Otto CM, Bonow RO, et al. 2014 AHA/ACC guideline for the management of patients with valvular heart disease. Circulation 2014;129:1–96.
8. Baurmgartner H, Falk V, Bax JJ, et al. 2017 ESC/EACTS guidelines for the management of valvular heart disease. Eur Heart J 2017;38(36):2739–91.
9. Pibarot P, Larose E, Dumesnil J. Imaging of valvular heart disease. Can J Cardiol 2013;29(3):337–49.
10. Nishimura RA, Otto CM, Bonow RO, et al. 2017 AHA/ACC focused update of the 2014 AHA/ACC guideline for the management of patients with valvular heart disease: a report of the American College of Cardiology/American Heart Association Task Force on Clinical Practice Guidelines. J Am Coll Cardiol 2017;70(2):252–89.
11. Kim M, Roman MJ, Cavallini C, et al. Effect of hypertension on aortic root size and prevalence of aortic regurgitation. Hypertension 1996;28:47–52.
12. Sapira JD. Quincke, de Musset, Duroziez, and Hill: some aortic regurgitation signs. South Med J 1981;74(4):459–67.
13. Gelfand EV, Hughes S, Hauser TH, et al. Severity of mitral and aortic regurgitation as assessed by cardiovascular magnetic resonance: optimizing correlation with Doppler echocardiography. J Cardiovasc Magn Reson 2006;8(3):503–7.
14. Faletra F, Pezzano A, Fusco R, et al. Measurement of mitral valve area in mitral stenosis: four echocardiographic methods compared with direct measurement of anatomic orifices. J Am Coll Cardiol 1996;28(5):1190–7.
15. Mirabel M, Iung B, Baron G, et al. What are the characteristics of patients with severe, symptomatic mitral regurgitation who are denied surgery? Eur Heart J 2007;28(11):1358–65.
16. Nishimura RA, Carabello BA, Faxon DP, et al. ACC/AHA 2008 Guideline update on valvular heart disease: focused update on infective endocarditis: a report of the American College of Cardiology/American Heart Association Task Force on Practice Guidelines endorsed by the Society of Cardiovascular Anesthesiologists, Society for Cardiovascular Angiography and Interventions, and Society of Thoracic Surgeons. J Am Coll Cardiol 2008;52(8):676–85.
17. Enriquez-Sarano M, Akins CW, Vahanian A. Mitral regurgitation. Lancet 2009; 9672:18–24.
18. Freed LA, Benjamin EJ, Levy D, et al. Mitral valve prolapse in the general population: the benign nature of echocardiographic features in the Framingham heart study. J Am Coll Cardiol 2002;40(7):1298–304.
19. Abhayaratna WP, Seward JB, Appleton CP, et al. Left atrial size: physiologic determinants and clinical applications. J Am Coll Cardiol 2006;47(2):2357–63.

20. Espersen K, Jensen EW, Rosenborg D, et al. Comparison of cardiac output measurement techniques: thermodilution, Doppler, CO2-rebreathing and the direct Fick method. Acta Anaesthesiol Scand 1995;39(2):245–51.
21. Delahaye JP, Gare JP, Viguier E, et al. Natural history of severe mitral regurgitation. Eur Heart J 1991;12(Supp B):5–9.
22. Bonow RO, Carabello BA, Chatterjee K, et al. 2008 focused update incorporated into the ACC/AHA 2006 guidelines for the management of patients with valvular heart disease: a report of the American College of Cardiology/American Heart Association Task Force on Practice Guidelines (Writing Committee to revise the 1998 guidelines for the management of patients with valvular heart disease). Endorsed by the Society of Cardiovascular Anesthesiologists, Society for Cardiovascular Angiography and Interventions, and Society of Thoracic Surgeons. J Am Coll Cardiol 2008;52(13):e1–142.
23. Steinberg BA, Piccini JP. Anticoagulation in atrial fibrillation. BMJ 2014;348: g2116.

Preparticipation Screening of Young Athletes

Identifying Cardiovascular Disease

Kyle P. Lammlein, MD[a],*, Jonathan M. Stoddard, MD[a],
Francis G. O'Connor, MD, MPH[b]

KEYWORDS

- Preparticipation physical examination • Cardiovascular screening
- Sudden cardiac death • ECG • Sports physical • Athlete's heart

KEY POINTS

- A major goal of the preparticipation physical examination (PPE) is to prevent sudden cardiac death in young athletes. This has proven to be difficult because many sudden cardiac deaths in young athletes are "unexplained."
- Highly trained athletes may develop physiologic cardiovascular changes that can sometimes result in abnormal electrocardiogram (ECG) tracings and borderline echocardiographic findings ("athlete's heart").
- The PPE should include the American Heart Association 14-element preparticipation cardiovascular screening checklist.
- There is insufficient evidence to recommend screening ECGs and echocardiograms for all young athletes during PPEs.
- Providers should be aware of the American Heart Association and American College of Cardiology recommendations for further evaluation when abnormal findings arise during the PPE.

INTRODUCTION: NATURE OF THE PROBLEM

The preparticipation physical examination (PPE), or sports physical examination, is an encounter familiar to most primary care physicians. Each year in the United States, thousands of children and young adults undergo PPEs, to screen for conditions that may be life threatening or disabling. Given recurrent, high-profile cases, a common

Disclosure Statement: The authors have no financial disclosures. The views expressed in this article are those of the authors and do not reflect the official policy or position of the Uniformed Services University, the Department of Defense, or the US Government.
[a] Family Medicine, National Capital Consortium Family Medicine Residency, Fort Belvoir Community Hospital, 9300 DeWitt Loop, Fort Belvoir, VA 22060, USA; [b] Department of Military and Emergency Medicine, Uniformed Services University of the Health Sciences, 4301 Jones Bridge Road, Bethesda, MD 20814, USA
* Corresponding author.
E-mail address: kyle.p.lammlein.mil@mail.mil

question physicians face is how best to screen for conditions that predispose young athletes to sudden cardiac death (SCD). Cardiovascular disorders account for nearly 75% of all sudden deaths in athletes.[1] Estimates of SCD rates in high school– and college-age athletes range from as high as 1:75,000 to 1:300,000.[2–4] Currently, there are no universally agreed upon standards to clear young athletes for sports participation. There remains considerable controversy in the sports medicine community as to what constitutes adequate cardiac screening. The use of ECG and echocardiography as screening tools are ongoing topics of debate. In addition, despite the broad implementation of routine PPE across the country, there has been little, if any, impact on the overall morbidity and mortality in young athletes.[5] This article explores current guidelines and controversies in preparticipation screening.

Overview of Athlete's Heart

It can be difficult to distinguish between normal physiologic changes (also known as athlete's heart or athletic heart syndrome) and pathologic cardiac changes.[6] This complicates the ability to accurately assess cardiovascular risk in athletes. Exercise of sufficient quantity and intensity can cause structural and electrical changes in the heart.[6] Endurance and strength training athletes have different cardiac adaptations as a result of sustained volume and pressure loads.[6] Intense endurance exercise can induce increased ventricular dilation and biventricular eccentric hypertrophy.[6] Pressure loads associated with strength training, in contrast, tend to cause concentric ventricular hypertrophy.[6] Eccentric hypertrophy is symmetric chamber dilation and wall thickening caused by repetitive ventricular stretching to increases cardiac output.[7,8] Concentric hypertrophy refers to significant wall thickening with little to no ventricular chamber dilation caused by repetitive sharp increases in blood pressure during strength training.[7] In the setting of concentric hypertrophy, increased contractility occurs without ventricular dilation.[7]

Exercise can also induce electrical changes in the heart. These electrical changes in the athlete's heart are primarily due to 1 of 2 causes. First, with training, a gradual response to catecholamines and increased parasympathetic tone leads to a decreased resting heart rate.[6] As a result of chamber dilation and hypertrophy, cardiac output is maintained at a lower heart rate. Second, electrical changes can occur as a result of the structural changes associated with both concentric and eccentric hypertrophy (**Boxes 1–3**).[6,9] In

---

Box 1
Normal electrocardiogram findings in the athlete (no further workup required)

Increased QRS voltage for left ventricular hypertrophy (LVH) or right ventricular hypertrophy (RVH)

Incomplete right bundle branch block (RBBB)

Early repolarization/ST segment elevation

ST elevation followed by T-wave inversion V1–V4 in black athletes

T-wave inversion V1–V3 age less than 16 years old

Sinus bradycardia or arrhythmia

Ectopic atrial or junctional rhythm

First-degree atrioventricular (AV) block

Mobitz type I second-degree AV block

Data from Drezner JA, Sharma S, Baggish A, et al. International criteria for electrocardiographic interpretation in athletes: consensus statement. Br J Sports Med 2017;51(9):704–31.

Box 2
Borderline electrocardiogram findings in the athlete (may consider further workup, especially if >1 finding)

Left-axis deviation

Left-atrial enlargement

Right-axis deviation

Right-atrial enlargement

Complete RBBB

Data from Drezner JA, Sharma S, Baggish A, et al. International criteria for electrocardiographic interpretation in athletes: consensus statement. Br J Sports Med 2017;51(9):704–31.

---

addition, although training can enhance parasympathetic tone and lead to a resting bradycardia, no change in maximal heart rate occurs with exercise training.

These adaptive structural and physiologic responses of the normal athletic heart to training do not rule out the possibility of a coexistent, underlying abnormality. This makes diagnosing cardiovascular disease in athletes that much more challenging because changes may present with overlapping features. Criteria to distinguish the characteristics of athletic heart syndrome from significant underlying abnormality have been defined.[9] There are a wide range of potential electrocardiographic (ECG) changes present in athletes (see **Boxes 1–3**). A study of highly trained elite athletes

---

Box 3
Abnormal electrocardiogram findings in the athlete (further workup required)

T-wave inversion

ST segment depression

Pathologic Q waves

Complete left bundle branch block

QRS $\geq$140 ms duration

Epsilon wave

Ventricular preexcitation

Prolonged QT interval

Brugada type 1 pattern

Profound sinus bradycardia less than 30 bpm

PR interval $\geq$400 ms

Mobitz type II 2° AV block

3° AV block

$\geq$2 Premature ventricular contractions

Atrial tachyarrhythmias

Ventricular arrhythmias

Data from Drezner JA, Sharma S, Baggish A, et al. International criteria for electrocardiographic interpretation in athletes: consensus statement. Br J Sports Med 2017;51(9):704–31.

suggests that there is no consistent correlation between ECG abnormalities and abnormal findings on echocardiography.[10]

Overview of Sudden Cardiac Death

SCD is defined as an unexpected natural death that is atraumatic, nonviolent, and of cardiac origin, occurring in an individual without a prior knowledge of an underlying (potentially fatal) cardiovascular disorder. The event generally occurs during or immediately following exercise.[11] Several high-profile cases have vaulted SCD into the public consciousness in recent years.[3] The overall rate of SCD is low, estimated at 1:75,000 to 1:300,000 young athletes per year.[2,3] The incidence is higher in male athletes (9:1).[12] Overall, male basketball and football players account for 50% to 61% of all identified cases of SCD, with the highest reported incidence among male college basketball players (1:9000 per year). African American athletes have the highest incidence of any race (1:21,000).[5,13] The reasons for this increased risk are not clear.

Although most data come from young, highly trained athletes, SCD is not limited to this demographic. The absolute number of SCD events is likely higher in the larger population of young individuals who do not compete in organized athletics.[3] This observation impacts the ongoing debate about approaches to screening.

In patients with underlying cardiac disease, exercise precipitates SCD.[5] For athletes less than 35 years of age, most events have historically been attributed to a ventricular tachyarrhythmia. To date, the most commonly hypothesized cause of SCD in young athletes has been hypertrophic cardiomyopathy (HCM; 30%–35%) followed by congenital coronary artery anomalies (15%–20%).[3] Other identified disorders are identified in **Box 4**, each of which accounts for less than 5% of SCD causes.[3] A

Box 4
Common causes of sudden cardiac death in young athletes

Hypertrophic cardiomyopathy (30%–35%)

Congenital coronary artery anomalies (15%–20%)

Arrhythmogenic right ventricular cardiomyopathy/dysplasia (<5%)

Myocarditis (<5%)

Valvular heart disease (<5%)

Dilated cardiomyopathy (<5%)

Premature atherosclerotic disease (<5%)

Congenital heart disease (<5%)

Wolf-Parkinson-White preexcitation (2%–3%)

Ion channelopathies (long QT syndrome, Brugada syndrome, catecholaminergic polymorphic ventricular tachycardia) (2%–3%)

Sickle cell trait (2%–3%)

Marfan syndrome (<5%)

Asthma (frequency undefined)

Pulmonary embolus (frequency undefined)

Ruptured cerebral aneurysm (frequency undefined)

Heat stroke (frequency undefined)

Performance enhancing or recreational drug use (frequency undefined)

nonarrhythmogenic mechanism of SCD is Marfan syndrome. In patients with Marfan syndrome, aortic dilation leads to aortic dissection or rupture and SCD. Other reported noncardiac causes of sudden death in young athletes include asthma, pulmonary embolus, ruptured cerebral aneurysm, heat stroke, and performance-enhancing or recreational drug use.[3]

A recent analysis of autopsy reports from SCD cases in National Collegiate Athletic Association athletes from 2003 to 2013 has cast doubt on the traditional mechanisms of SCD. In this series, autopsy-negative sudden unexplained death was the most common finding (25%).[13] Definitive evidence of HCM was found in only 8% of autopsies.[13] Data from the Department of Defense Cardiovascular Death Registry reported sudden unexplained death in 41% of service members less than 35 years of age. HCM was reported in only 13% of cases.[14] In athletes older than 35, defined unsuspected atherosclerotic coronary artery disease is the leading cause of SCD.[12]

THE CARDIOVASCULAR PREPARTICIPATION EVALUATION

One of the primary objectives of the PPE is to ensure safe participation in athletics by identifying those at risk for poor outcomes due to preexisting, clinically relevant abnormalities.[12] Because cardiovascular abnormalities are difficult to detect, a standardized set of history questions and physical examination techniques has been created to optimize the utility of the preparticipation evaluation.[2] The American Heart Association (AHA) has developed a standardized 14-element approach to screen competitive athletes (**Boxes 5** and **6**). This comprehensive evaluation includes items from the patient's personal history, family history, and physical examination.[3] A positive response

---

Box 5
Medical history portion (items 1–10) of American Heart Association 14-element preparticipation cardiovascular screening

Personal history

1. Chest pain, discomfort, tightness, or pressure related to exertion

2. Unexplained syncope/near-syncope that is judged not to be vasovagal in origin

3. Excessive and unexplained dyspnea, fatigue, or palpitations associated with exercise

4. Prior recognition of a heart murmur

5. Elevated systemic blood pressure

6. Prior restriction from participation in sports

7. Prior testing of the heart, ordered by a physician

Family history

8. Premature death (sudden and unexpected, or otherwise) before 50 years of age attributable to heart disease in $\geq$1 relative

9. Disability from heart disease in a close relative less than 50 years of age

10. Hypertrophic or dilated cardiomyopathy, long QT syndrome, or other ion channelopathies, Marfan syndrome, or clinically significant arrhythmias; specific knowledge of genetic cardiac conditions in family members

Adapted from Maron BJ, Friedman RA, Kligfield P, et al. Assessment of the 12-lead ECG as a screening test for detection of cardiovascular disease in healthy general populations of young people (12–25 years of age): a scientific statement from the American Heart Association and the American College of Cardiology. Circulation 2014;130:1305.

> **Box 6**
> **Physical examination portion (items 11–14) of American Heart Association 14-element preparticipation cardiovascular screening**
>
> *Physical examination*
>
> 1. Auscultation for heart murmurs
>
> 2. Palpation of femoral and radial pulses to exclude aortic coarctation
>
> 3. Observation for physical stigmata of Marfan syndrome
>
> 4. Brachial artery blood pressure measurement
>
> *Adapted from* Maron BJ, Friedman RA, Kligfield P, et al. Assessment of the 12-lead ECG as a screening test for detection of cardiovascular disease in healthy general populations of young people (12–25 years of age): a scientific statement from the American Heart Association and the American College of Cardiology. Circulation 2014;130:1305.

or finding prompts referral for additional cardiovascular evaluation.[12] The initial evaluation should be conducted between 12 and 14 years age and then repeated every 1 to 3 years. Screening should occur before the start of the sports season to allow for secondary testing to be completed if necessary. Unfortunately, fewer than 50% of primary care physicians are aware of the current AHA recommendations.[5]

Patient History

The first 10 elements of the screening evaluation are based on a targeted personal and family medical history (see **Box 5**).[15] Parental verification of historical data is highly recommended for athletes in high school and middle school.[3] This clinical history detects more abnormalities than the physical examination and is also more likely to prompt physicians to restrict athletic participation.[2] A critical symptom is exertional syncope. Exertional syncope is a distinct event that is often unrecognized and is an ominous sign of underlying cardiovascular disease.[16] The evaluating physician must, therefore, distinguish between true syncope (involving a loss of consciousness and presumed hemodynamic compromise) and exercise-associated collapse (associated with exhaustive effort or postexercise hypotension). The postevent state provides other clues as to the cause of syncope as does reports from individuals witnessing the event. In true syncope from hemodynamic causes, unless resuscitation is required, the athlete typically recovers quickly with restoration of arterial pressure. Collapse following an exhaustive effort is generally associated with more prolonged periods of disorientation, even in the supine position with normal heart rate and blood pressure. Patients with syncope due to heat stress are universally hypotensive and tachycardic. Athletes with heat stroke have an elevated core temperature and mental status changes. Athletes who are able to assist in their own evacuation are unlikely to suffer from a life-threatening arrhythmia, although other metabolic abnormalities are possible (eg, hyponatremia).

The second critical distinction is whether the event occurred during or immediately after exercise. Orthostatic hypotension occurring after exercise and the sudden cessation of activity is much less ominous than a sudden loss of consciousness occurring during exercise, which suggests an arrhythmogenic cause. Syncope prompted by an abrupt loud noise (such as a starting gun) or immersion in cold water may suggest long QT syndrome (LQTS). Seizure activity can be the result of reduced cerebral perfusion and therefore does not necessarily always imply epilepsy. Incontinence suggests seizure activity. Vital signs (including body temperature) may suggest heat injury.

A detailed assessment of events before the collapse provides additional information about potential causes. Prodromal symptoms such as palpitations (suggesting arrhythmia), chest pain (ischemia, aortic dissection), nausea (ischemia or high levels of vagal activity), wheezing, and pruritus (anaphylaxis) suggest certain conditions. It is important to note whether symptoms occur only during exercise, or if there are other precipitating events. It is important to identify whether syncope occurs only in the upright position (orthostatic hypotension) or also sitting or supine (arrhythmia or non-hemodynamic cause).

The next component of the historical evaluation assesses for medication and supplement use. A comprehensive medication list includes over-the-counter medications and performance-enhancing supplements. The practice of high-risk behaviors, such as recreational drug use, should be elucidated as well. Finally, a personal and family history of sudden death helps to identify very-high-risk subgroups with HCM, LQTS, or right ventricular cardiomyopathy.

Physical Examination

Items 11 through 14 of the screening evaluation focus on a targeted physical examination (see **Box 6**). The physical examination should be conducted in an environment that allows for optimal auscultation of the heart.[12] Auscultation should be performed with the patient in both the supine and the standing position.[3] Dynamic auscultation should be performed by using the Valsalva and squat-to-stand maneuvers. These maneuvers help to identify the type of murmur and to augment previously inaudible murmurs. The squatting maneuver increases stroke volume, whereas standing and the Valsalva maneuver lead to decreased stroke volume. Most murmurs will become louder with squatting (increased stroke volume) and softer with standing or Valsalva (decreased stroke volume). Murmurs that become softer with squatting and louder with standing or Valsalva raise the suspicion for HCM or mitral valve prolapse.[2]

Well-conditioned athletes have predictable changes in the cardiovascular examination. For example, because of enhanced vagal tone, decreased resting sympathetic tone, and a larger stroke volume, well-conditioned athletes often exhibit a resting bradycardia (between 40 and 60 bpm). Sinus bradycardia is common among trained athletes, and sinus arrhythmia may be more noticeable. The physiologic splitting of S2 may also be slightly delayed during inspiration because of the larger stroke volume. An S3 may be noted in endurance-trained athletes secondary to the increased rate of left ventricular filling associated with the relative left ventricular dilatation.[2,17] Although an S4 may be normal in strength-trained athletes (because of concentric hypertrophy), detection always warrants further evaluation. Functional (flow) murmurs are often present when supine and diminished with standing or Valsalva and may be noted in up to 30% to 50% of athletes on careful examination.[18]

Palpation of the femoral pulses with simultaneous palpation of the radial pulse screens for coarctation of the aorta. Delay (or decreased intensity) of the femoral pulse compared with the radial pulse (radiofemoral delay) suggests coarctation and warrants further evaluation.[2] Evaluating for the stigmata of Marfan syndrome helps identify athletes at risk for aortic root dilatation and sudden death secondary to aortic dissection. There currently is no evidence based guidance for appropriate screening for Marfan syndrome or other connective tissue disorders, but current diagnostic criteria and the PPE monograph provides some guidance for clinical consideration.[19,20] The most important historical information is a family history of Marfan syndrome, and personal history of early childhood myopia. Physical examination signs of Marfan syndrome that should raise concern for a potential connective disorder include: the thumb sign (entire nail of the thumb projects beyond the ulnar border of the hand when hand is clenched without assistance); the wrist sign (thumb overlaps distal interphalangeal joint of fifth finger when hand is wrapped around opposite wrist); arm span greater than body height, high-arched palate; arachnodactyly (long, spidery fingers); pectus excavatum; lenticular dislocation; myopia; mitral valve prolapse; aortic insufficiency murmur; and kyphosis.[19] Patients with a family history of Marfan Syndrome or 2 or more clinical manifestations suggesting a connective tissue disorder should be further evaluated with resting ECG, slit-lamp eye examination, and echocardiography.[2]

Measurement of blood pressure should be performed with the patient in the sitting position and the arm well supported at heart level. Measurements should ideally be taken in both arms.[3] Blood pressure readings for pediatric patients should be interpreted and managed based on guidelines provided by the National Heart, Lung, and Blood Institute Expert Panel on Integrated Guidelines for Cardiovascular Health and Risk Reduction in Children and Adolescents.[21] Blood pressure readings for adult patients should be interpreted and managed based on guidelines provided by the Eighth Joint National Committee.[22]

Table 1 lists additional correlations between common causes of SCD and their respective history and physical examination findings.

IMAGING AND ADDITIONAL TESTING

A growing area of interest and controversy in sports medicine is the addition of screening ECG as part of the routine PPE. There are significant data in support of screening ECGs to decrease SCD rates due to increased detection of certain cardiac conditions associated with SCD.[5] A recent Italian study showed that universal screening ECGs on young athletes aged 12 to 35 reduced SCD rates by 90% in a 2-year period.[3] An estimated 60% of the disorders associated with SCD in young athletes may have ECG abnormalities identifiable to professionals with considerable ECG interpretation experience.[5] False positive rates of screening ECGs can range as low as 3% to 6% in centers with experienced clinicians using modern interpretation standards.[5]

Arguments against routine screening ECG suggest that although universal screening would increase the detection of some cardiac disorders that could lead to SCD, there is the potential that (1) ECG evidence of disease is not present on day of test, (2) the abnormality is missed by interpreter, or (3) patient has cardiac disease without ECG changes.[5] The ECG is not a perfect screening test for conditions that cause SCD. The previously mentioned Italian study has several important limitations. First, it was applied to a population with a higher prevalence of SCD in young athletes (4.3/100,000 in Italy vs 0.5–1.3 in the United States).[3] In addition, the most common cause of SCD in young athletes in the Italian study was arrhythmogenic right ventricular cardiomyopathy/dysplasia.[3] Early-onset coronary artery disease was also common in this region, whereas HCM was relatively uncommon.[3] This is in contrast to the US population, whereby these conditions are much less common and HCM is, by far, the most common identified cause of SCD in the young athlete.[2,3,5] Because of these differences, it is unclear whether a similar ECG screening program in the United States would produce the same results. Cost is an additional concern because it would take an estimated $2 billion to implement an annual screening program.[3] This equates to an estimated $14 million per case identified.[3] The feasibility of screening around 10 million young athletes across the United States with screening ECGs, ensuring competent, consistent interpretations as well as prompt and practical follow-up

Table 1
Common causes of sudden death in young athletes with associated history and physical examination findings

Condition	History Features	Physical Examination Findings
HCM	Family history of HCM, premature sudden death, recurrent syncope, or lethal arrhythmias requiring urgent treatment. Personal history of exertional chest pain or syncope	Wide range of auscultatory findings, from normal examination to a harsh midsystolic murmur that accentuates with standing or the Valsalva maneuver
Coronary artery disease (congenital or acquired)	Family history of early coronary artery disease, premature sudden death, or coronary anomalies. Personal history of exercise-induced chest pain, syncope, or fatigue	Usually normal
Marfan syndrome	Family history of Marfan syndrome or premature sudden death	See "Physical Examination" section.
LQTS	Family history of premature sudden death. Personal history of palpitations or recurrent syncope	Unremarkable
Brugada syndrome (genetic disorder of myocardial sodium ion channels)	Family history of premature sudden death, particularly in men of Southeast Asian descent	Unremarkable
Myocarditis	Personal history of fatigue, exertional dyspnea, syncope, palpitations, arrhythmias, or acute congestive heart failure	May be normal. Palpable or auscultated extra systoles, third or fourth heart sound gallops, and other clinical signs of heart failure should be considered suspicious
Arrhythmogenic right ventricular cardiomyopathy	Family history of premature sudden death; more common in persons of Mediterranean descent. Personal history of palpitations or recurrent syncope	Unremarkable
Aortic stenosis	Personal history of exercise-induced chest pain, breathlessness, light-headedness, syncope, or dizziness	Constant apical ejection click; harsh systolic ejection murmur heard best at the upper right sternal border; crescendo-decrescendo murmur, normally grade 3 murmur or higher

testing is very challenging. In addition, some studies point to higher rates of SCD in nonathletes, leading to the question of implementing ECG screening for all persons aged 12 to 35 (an estimated 60 million patients), making the feasibility of universal screening unlikely.[3]

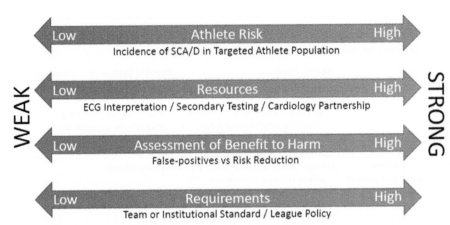

Fig. 1. Strength of rationale for ECG screening. SCA/D, Sudden cardiac arrest and death. (*From* Drezner JA, O'Connor FG, Harmon KG, et al. AMSSM position statement on cardiovascular preparticipation screening in athletes: current evidence, knowledge gaps, recommendations and future directions. Br J Sports Med 2017;51:163; with permission.)

Currently, most professional organizations recommend against universal screening. The AHA, American Academy of Family Physicians, American Medical Society for Sports Medicine (AMSSM), and National Institutes of Health do not support a universal ECG program as part of the PPE.[2,3,5] The AMSSM has recently recommended that clinicians use their best medical judgment based on their evaluation to determine whether an ECG is warranted as a part of the PPE[5] (**Fig. 1**).

Box 7
American Heart Association/American College of Cardiology task forces

Task Force 1: Classification of sport: dynamic, static, and impact

Task Force 2: Preparticipation screening for cardiovascular disease in competitive athletes

Task Force 3: Hypertrophic cardiomyopathy, arrhythmogenic right ventricular cardiomyopathy and other cardiomyopathies, and myocarditis

Task Force 4: Congenital heart disease

Task Force 5: Valvular heart disease

Task Force 6: Hypertension

Task Force 7: Aortic diseases, including Marfan syndrome

Task Force 8: Coronary artery disease

Task Force 9: Arrhythmias and conduction defects

Task Force 10: The cardiac channelopathies

Task Force 11: Drugs and performance-enhancing substances

Task Force 12: Emergency action plans, resuscitation, cardiopulmonary resuscitation, and automated external defibrillators

Task Force 13: Commotio cordis

Task Force 14: Sickle cell trait

Task Force 15: Legal aspects of medical eligibility and disqualification recommendations

An additional proposal for universal screening in the United States includes the use of transthoracic echocardiography (TTE). This screening method is far more sensitive and specific for detecting HCM, the most common known cause of SCD in American athletes. TTE is not currently recommended for screening in young athletes because of its relative high cost and lack of feasibility for universal screening.[2] TTE is also limited by the difficulty presented by overlapping features of the athletic heart syndrome and pathologic heart disease. Because of these issues, TTE is not currently recommended as a screening tool. It is useful, however, as part of a more comprehensive evaluation when abnormal findings on PPE or ECG are identified.[3]

CARDIAC CLEARANCE FOR PARTICIPATION

The AHA and American College of Cardiology have recently provided expert guidance on eligibility and disqualification parameters for young athletes if abnormal findings arise during the PPE.[23] This resource classifies cardiac disorders that may require scrutiny before permitting clearance to specific sports into 15 task forces (**Box 7**). *Preparticipation Physical Evaluation, 4th edition* is another useful resource for routine use by all physicians conducting routine PPE.[22] This resource discusses the PPE in complete detail, highlights indications for further workup, and makes recommendations about clearance for participation based on findings from the PPE.[22] Because of the high number of cardiac diagnoses and variations of symptoms and clinical findings in each, there exists no succinct list of absolute disqualifying diagnoses.[22] *Preparticipation Physical Evaluation* makes specific recommendations for continued play (often given specific recommendations based on what sport is being played) based on diagnosis, symptoms, and clinical findings.[22]

SUMMARY

The goal of the PPE is to detect risk factors for SCD, make risk-based decisions regarding further workup, and ultimately recommend for or against participation. The PPE is a complex and evolving area of interest among sports medicine physicians. Current evidence suggests that the most common cause of SCD in young US athletes is unknown. Despite these challenges, experts from numerous medical organizations recommend annual PPEs before athletic participation. The AHA 14-element preparticipation cardiovascular screening tool is commonly recommended. Universal screening of young athletes with ECGs and echocardiograms is not currently recommended in the United States. There is an emerging shift toward targeted, risk-based approaches to identify which individual athletes would benefit from ECG or echocardiography. Providers should continue to use clinical judgment for each individual patient in determining if any further testing is indicated.

REFERENCES

1. Harmon KG, Asif IM, Klossner D, et al. Incidence of sudden cardiac death in National Collegiate Athletic Association athletes. Circulation 2011;123:1594–600.
2. Giese EA, O'Connor FG, Brennan FH, et al. The athletic preparticipation evaluation: cardiovascular assessment. Am Fam Physician 2007;75(7):1008–14.
3. Maron BJ, Friedman RA, Kligfield P, et al. Assessment of the 12-lead ECG as a screening test for detection of cardiovascular disease in healthy general populations of young people (12-25 years of age): a scientific statement

from the American Heart Association and the American College of Cardiology. Circulation 2014;130:1303–34.

4. O'Connor FG, Oriscello RP. Cardiovascular considerations in the athlete. Chapter 53. In: Birrer RB, O'Connor FG, Oriscello RP, editors. Musculoskeletal and sports medicine: essentials for the primary care practitioner. 4th edition. Boca Raton (FL): CRC Press; 2015. p. 631–44.

5. Drezner JA, O'Connor FG, Harmon KG, et al. AMSSM position statement on cardiovascular preparticipation screening in athletes: current evidence, knowledge gaps, recommendations and future directions. Br J Sports Med 2017;51:153–67.

6. Lauschke J, Maisch B. Athlete's heart or hypertrophic cardiomyopathy? Clin Res Cardiol 2009;98:80–8.

7. Mihl C, Dassen WR, Kuipers H. Cardiac remodelling: concentric versus eccentric hypertrophy in strength and endurance athletes. Neth Heart J 2008;16:129–33.

8. Fagard R. Athlete's heart. Heart 2003;89(12):1455–61.

9. Drezner JA, Sharma S, Baggish A, et al. International criteria for electrocardiographic interpretation in athletes: consensus statement. Br J Sports Med 2017; 51(9):704–31.

10. Pelliccia A, Maron BJ, Spataro A, et al. The upper limit of physiologic cardiac hypertrophy in highly trained elite athletes. N Engl J Med 1991;324:295–301.

11. Pigozzi F, Rizzo M. Sudden death in competitive athletes. Clinic Sports Med 2008;27:153–81.

12. Maron BJ, Thompson PD, Ackerman MJ, et al. Recommendations and considerations related to preparticipation screening for cardiovascular abnormalities in competitive athletes: 2007 update. A scientific statement from the American Heart Association Council on Nutrition, Physical Activity, and Metabolism: endorsed by the American College of Cardiology Foundation. Circulation 2007; 115:1643–55.

13. Harmon KG, Asif IM, Maleszewski JJ, et al. Incidence, etiology, and comparative frequency of sudden cardiac death in NCAA athletes: a decade in review. American Heart Association. Circulation 2015;132(1):10–9.

14. Eckart RE, Shry EA, Burke AP, et al. Sudden death in young adults: an autopsy-based series of a population undergoing active surveillance. J Am Coll Cardiol 2011;58:1254–61.

15. Childress MA, O'Connor FG, Levine BD. Exertional collapse in the runner: evaluation and management in fieldside and office-based settings. Clin Sports Med 2010;29(3):459–76.

16. Drezner JA, Fudge J, Harmon KG, et al. Warning symptoms and family history in children and young adults with sudden cardiac arrest. J Am Board Fam Med 2012;25(4):408–15.

17. Mukerji B, Alpert MA, Mukerji V. Cardiovascular changes in athletes. Am Fam Physician 1989;40:169–75.

18. Huston TP, Puffer JC, Rodney WM. The athletic heart syndrome. N Engl J Med 1985;313:24–32.

19. Bernhardt DT, Roberts WO. Preparticipation physical evaluation. 4th edition. Elk Grove Village (IL): American Academy of Pediatrics; 2010.

20. Summers KM, West JA, Hattam A, et al. Recent developments in the diagnosis of Marfan syndrome and related disorders. Med J Aust 2012;197(9):494–7.

21. Daniels SR, Benuck I, Christakis DA, et al. Expert panel on integrated guidelines for cardiovascular health and risk reduction in children and adolescents: summary report. Bethesda, (MD): U.S. Department of Health and

Human Services. National Heart, Lung, and Blood Institute; 2012. NIH Publication No. 12-7486A.

22. James PA, Oparil S, Carter BL, et al. 2014 evidence-based guideline for the management of high blood pressure in adults report from the panel members appointed to the eighth Joint National Committee (JNC 8). JAMA 2014;311(5): 507–20.

23. Maron BJ, Zipes DP, Kovacs RJ, on behalf of the American Heart Association Electrocardiography and Arrhythmias Committee of the Council on Clinical Cardiology, Council on Cardiovascular Disease in the Young, Council on Cardiovascular and Stroke Nursing, Council on Functional Genomics and Translational Biology, and the American College of Cardiology. Eligibility and disqualification recommendations for competitive athletes with cardiovascular abnormalities: preamble, principles, and general considerations: a scientific statement from the American Heart Association and American College of Cardiology. Circulation 2015;132:e256–61.

Metabolic Syndrome
Systems Thinking in Heart Disease

Ron Dommermuth, MD[a],*, Kristine Ewing, MD[b]

KEYWORDS

- Metabolic syndrome • Insulin resistance • Diabetes prevention • Ectopic obesity

KEY POINTS

- Metabolic syndrome (MetS) is a cluster of risk factors that contribute to the development of type 2 diabetes mellitus and atherosclerotic disease.
- MetS is a progressive, pathophysiologic state of interrelated risk factors increasingly resistant to treatment over time. Ectopic obesity, dietary sugar, insulin resistance, and inflammation contribute significantly.
- Uric acid, inflammatory markers, and bioactive adipokines contribute pathophysiologically and may become useful clinical markers for identifying and managing MetS.
- Clinical phenotypes (adiposity, vascular, lipid, insulin resistant, and hormonal dominant) and staging have been described and can translate to specific evidence-based treatment.
- Treatment must include, but not be limited to, therapeutic lifestyle change.

INTRODUCTION

Metabolic syndrome (MetS) is a major public health concern through the substantial role it contributes to the incidence of type 2 diabetes mellitus (T2DM) and atherosclerotic cardiovascular disease (CVD.) MetS is currently defined by the presence of 3 of 5 of the following criteria: abdominal obesity (waist circumference >102 in [men] or 88 in [women]), atherogenic dyslipidemia: serum triglycerides (TG) greater than 150 mg/dL or serum high-density lipoprotein (HDL) less than 40 mg/dl (men) or less than 50 mg/dL (women), elevated blood pressure (BP) (>130/85 mm Hg), or insulin

Disclosure Statement: No competing financial interests exist. This research did not receive any specific grant from funding agencies in the public, commercial, or not-for-profit sectors. The views expressed in this article are those of the authors and do not necessarily reflect the official policy or position of the Department of the Navy, Department of Defense, or the US Government.
[a] Northwest Washington Family Medicine Residency, 2512 Wheaton Way, Suite B, Bremerton, WA 98310, USA; [b] Department of Family Medicine, Naval Hospital Bremerton, 1 Boone Road, Bremerton, WA 98312, USA
* Corresponding author.
E-mail address: ronald.dommermuth@harrisonmedical.org

resistance with impaired fasting glucose (or drug treatment of hyperglycemia). The prevalence of MetS in the United States approaches 30%. Among obese individuals, the incidence is as high as 65%.[1,2]

The pathogenesis of MetS is complex and is more than a sum of its component parts (obesity, atherogenic dyslipidemia, hypertension, and insulin resistance). From a systems perspective, MetS is a progressive, interdependent pathophysiologic state composed of causally interrelated risk factors that become increasingly resistant to treatment as the condition progresses. Ectopic (especially liver and muscle) and visceral obesity, inflammation, insulin resistance, and dietary sugar consumption play key roles in disease pathogenesis. MetS seems to be a transgenerational nongenetic disorder because the metabolic state of the mother during each pregnancy programs fetal metabolism to establish a trajectory toward future obesity.[3,4]

Although medical and surgical therapies are useful adjuncts in managing MetS, lifestyle change is the cornerstone of treatment. From a systems perspective, initiatives at the individual, community, and national levels are necessary to combat MetS.

COMMON CLINICAL SCENARIOS

The following are common presentations of MetS in primary care:

Case 1: a 43-year-old man presenting with a new diagnosis of gouty arthritis, body mass index (BMI) 35, abdominal waist circumference 102 cm in, BP 138/88, elevated transaminases 1-times to 2-times normal, creatinine 1.3, total cholesterol 242 mg/dL, and High-density lipoprotein (HDL) 35 mg/dL. Prior abdominal imaging showed hepatic steatosis.

Case 2: a 33-year-old woman with BMI 32. Her history includes gestational diabetes with glucose intolerance on subsequent testing and a normal lipid profile. She presents with complaints of oligomenorrhea and she desires to conceive again.

Case 3: an 18-year-old woman with a velvety rash on her neck whose weight has crossed growth curve percentiles and now stands above the 95th percentile for age. Her total cholesterol is 400 mg/dL, HDL is 42 mg/dL, and fasting glucose is 101 mg/dL.

Case 4: a 28-year-old Hispanic woman presents for routine cytology screening. Her BMI is 27. She has a sedentary office job, does not exercise, and has a family history of obesity and T2DM.

DEFINITION

The definition of MetS remains the subject of debate (**Table 1**). Insulin resistance is generally agreed to be a central component. Controversy remains surrounding hyperglycemia thresholds, methods of obesity assessment (BMI vs waist circumference (WC, which is a more accurate predictor of ectopic visceral obesity)), and atherogenic dyslipidemia characterized by either elevated TG or suppression of HDL and elevated BP. Some investigators suggest adding inflammatory or prothrombotic markers, including C-reactive protein, interleukin 6, plasminogen activator inhibitor, insulin levels, uric acid levels, and microalbuminuria, to better reflect the underlying pathophysiology. Other investigators emphasize phenotypic features, such as polycystic ovary syndrome (PCOS), obstructive sleep apnea (OSA), chronic kidney disease, and fatty liver disease.[5] Population analyses have further identified racial phenotypic variability not reflected in existing criteria, suggesting the need to further adjust criteria for age and ethnicity.[6]

Table 1
Metabolic syndrome definition

Organization	Metabolic Syndrome Definition	Insulin Resistance or Hyperglycemia	Body Weight	Dyslipidemia	Elevated Blood Pressure	Other
World Health Organization (1998)	Insulin resistance + any other 2 criteria	Impaired glucose tolerance, impaired fasting glucose, or lowered insulin sensitivity	Men: waist-to-hip ratio >0.90 Women: waist-to-hip ratio >0.85 and/or BMI >30 kg/m^2	TG ≥150 mg/dL and/or HDL-C <35 mg/dL in men or <39 mg/dL in women	≥140/90 mm Hg	Microalbuminuria
European Group for the Study of Insulin Resistance (1999)	Insulin resistance + any other 2 criteria	Plasma insulin >75th percentile, impaired glucose tolerance, or impaired fasting glucose (but not diabetes)	WC ≥94 cm in men or ≥80 cm in women	TG ≥150 mg/dL and/or HDL-C <39 mg/dL in men or women	≥140/90 mm Hg or on therapy	None
Adult Treatment Panel III (2001)	Any 3 of 5 criteria	>110 mg/dL (modified in 2004 to >100 mg/dL), diabetes	WC ≥102 cm in men or ≥88 cm in women	TG ≥150 mg/dL, HDL-C <40 mg/dL in men or <50 mg/dL in women	≥130/85 mm Hg	None

(continued on next page)

Table 1
(continued)

Organization	Metabolic Syndrome Definition	Insulin Resistance or Hyperglycemia	Body Weight	Dyslipidemia	Elevated Blood Pressure	Other
American Association of Clinical Endocrinologists (2003)	Insulin resistance + any of the other criteria	Impaired glucose tolerance or impaired fasting glucose (but not diabetes)	BMI ≥25 kg/m^2	TG ≥150 mg/dL and HDL-C <40 mg/dL in men or <50 mg/dL in women	≥130/85 mm Hg	Other features of insulin resistance, including family history of diabetes, polycystic ovary syndrome, sedentary lifestyle, and so on
International Diabetes Federation (2005)	Body weight + any other 2 criteria	>100 mg/dL, diabetes	Increased WC (population specific)	TG ≥150 mg/dL or on therapy, HDL-C <40 mg/dL in men or <50 mg/dL in women or on therapy	≥130 mm Hg SBP or ≥85 mm Hg DBP or on therapy	None
American Heart Association/National Heart, Lung, and Blood Institute (2005)	Any 3 of 5 criteria	>100 mg/dL or on therapy	WC ≥102 cm in men or ≥88 cm in women	TG ≥150 mg/dL or on therapy, HDL-C <40 mg/dL in men or <50 mg/dL in women or on therapy	≥130 mm Hg SBP or ≥85 mm Hg DBP or on therapy	None

Abbreviations: HDL-C, HDL cholesterol; WC, waist circumference.
From Sperling LS, Mechanick JI, Neeland IJ, et al. The cardiometabolic health alliance working toward a new care model for the metabolic syndrome. J Am Coll Cardiol 2015;66(9):1055; with permission.

PATHOGENESIS

MetS results from a complex interplay of multiple external and intrinsic factors. Obesity, (in particular visceral obesity), plays an instigating role, whereas chronic inflammation and insulin resistance contribute to metabolic dysregulation.[7,8] Highlighting this association, the incidence of obesity mirrors that of MetS.[9] MetS is present in 5% of normal weight individuals, 22% of overweight individuals, and up to 65% obese individuals.[10,11]

Excess energy availability contributes to pathologic adiposity. Adipocyte function varies by site. Subcutaneous adipose is functionally different than ectopic or visceral obesity. Differential deposition of adipose tissue is influenced by modifiable factors (activity, nutritional status, growth hormone, and steroid levels) and nonmodifiable factors (gender, age, ethnicity, and genetic susceptibility). Whereas subcutaneous adipose can grow through cell size (hypertrophy) and cell number (hyperplasia), ectopic and visceral adipose are prone to hyperplasia and impaired function. Adipose tissue is an active endocrine organ that secretes bioactive adipokines. Adipokine secretion by ectopic and visceral adipose is dysfunctional and leads to free fatty acid elevation.[8] This, in turn, elevates TG levels, activating hepatic gluconeogenesis. The net result is hyperglycemia, TG synthesis, and overproduction of atherogenic very low-density lipoprotein particles.[12] Excess TGs deposited in ectopic tissue or visceral fat stores induce an inflammatory cascade resulting in a self-amplifying cytokine network. These dysfunctional ectopic adipocytes overexpress adipokines that promote insulin resistance while underproducing adiponectin and omentin-1, which normally act to reduce both chronic inflammation and insulin resistance and may be protective against cardiopulmonary injury.[5,13]

In addition, visceral obesity alters renal and splanchnic microcirculation leading to activation of the renin-angiotensin-aldosterone system and the sympathetic nervous system. This activation increases heart rate and sodium retention and alters endothelial and cardiac function.[14] Additionally, activated macrophages, over-represented in ectopic obesity, produce inflammatory cytokines, including tumor necrosis factor, interleukins 1 and 6, angiotensinogen, and plasminogen activator inhibitor. As an end result, these chronic metabolic and regulatory pathway alterations, including inappropriate hepatic glucose release, reduction in glucagon-like peptide function, and apancreatic B-cell dysfunction, lead to insulin resistance, inefficient protein synthesis, and chronic inflammation.[7,15] The pathologic role of ectopic obesity is further suggested by the existence of a metabolically healthy phenotypic variant of obesity. Obesity characterized by greater subcutaneous fat, lower visceral fat, and lower levels of circulating inflammatory markers.[16]

Insulin resistance contributes directly to hyperglycemia, elevated free fatty acids, hyperinsulinemia, and sympathetic nervous system activation. Under normal conditions pancreatic beta cells release insulin in response to increased serum glucose, which enhances glucose uptake and promotes normal adipogenesis by suppressing hepatic gluconeogenesis and lipolysis. In the insulin-resistant state, energy homeostasis is altered, resulting in inappropriate hepatic glucose production, reduced effectiveness of glucagon-like peptide, inefficient protein synthesis, and inadequate clearance of glycosylated end products,[15] resulting in cardiovascular system dysregulation, altered myocardial fuel substrate selection, microvascular dysfunction, accelerated coronary atherosclerosis, increased left ventricular mass, and cardiac diastolic dysfunction, ultimately increasing the risk for ischemia and heart failure.[14,17]

FRUCTOSE AND URIC ACID

Fructose is ubiquitous in the Western diet and in sugar-sweetened beverages (SSBs). Fructose does not induce the same level of insulin secretion as deos glucose. Fructose is rapidly absorbed by hepatocytes, stimulating unnecessary lipogenesis and further contributing to insulin resistance as well as visceral obesity.[15,18,19]

Elevated levels of uric acid are associated with and predict the development of hypertension and T2DM. Uric acid blocks insulin-mediated nitric oxide release, facilitates TG accumulation in hepatocytes, and inhibits adipocyte function, resulting in diminished levels of adiponectin (a cardioprotective adipokine). Hyperuricemia promotes microvascular and inflammatory changes in the kidney, resulting in enhanced salt sensitivity and hypertension. Hyperuricemia portends the development of T2DM, and studies have demonstrated a reduction in BP when uric acid is lowered therapeutically.[20,21]

METABOLIC SYNDROME PHENOTYPES AND STAGING

Multiple phenotypic subtypes of MetS have been described (**Fig. 1**), including adiposity dominant, insulin resistance dominant, vascular dominant, lipid dominant, and others.[2]

In the setting of MetS, the likelihood of adverse health consequences increases as risk factors accumulate, providing the basis for a proposed staging system (**Fig. 2**).[22]

Stage A includes those at risk for MetS but without any of the 5 defining criteria. Patients in stage B meet 1 or 2 criteria or have alternate risk factors. Stage C patients fully meet criteria but have yet to demonstrate end-organ damage, and stage D patients are defined by the presence of end-organ injury. This clinical staging system is useful in that it acknowledges the heterogeneity of MetS and prioritizes an absolute clinical risk assessment into the treatment plan.

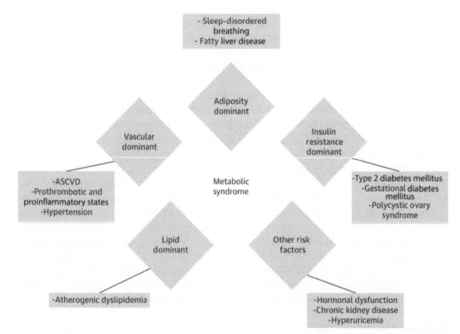

Fig. 1. MetS phenotypes. (*From* Sperling LS, Mechanick JI, Neeland IJ, et al. The cardiometabolic health alliance working toward a new care model for the metabolic syndrome. J Am Coll Cardiol 2015;66(9):1056; with permission.)

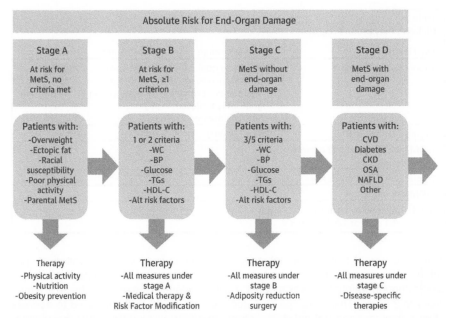

Fig. 2. MetS staging system. Alt, alternative; NAFLD, nonalcoholic fatty liver disease; WC, waist circumference. (*From* Sperling LS, Mechanick JI, Neeland IJ, et al. The cardiometabolic health alliance working toward a new care model for the metabolic syndrome. J Am Coll Cardiol 2015;66(9):1059; with permission.)

MANAGEMENT: TREATMENT GOALS IN METABOLIC SYNDROME

The management of MetS involves a multifaceted approach that is designed to stop weight gain, reverse overweight or obesity, normalize cardiovascular function, normalize insulin resistance and metabolic parameters, manage dyslipidemia, and prevent (or treat) end-organ disease. Lifestyle changes are the cornerstone for stopping or reversing disease.

Lifestyle Changes

Lifestyle changes are difficult to sustain. The Diabetes Prevention Program (DPP) trial defined essential elements of lifestyle change for individuals at risk of MetS (**Table 2**). Essential components of lifestyle changes described by the DPP include a target goal of 7% weight loss; a low-calorie, low-fat diet; and 150 minutes of moderate exercise per week (ie, brisk walking).[23]

Among those without MetS at baseline, lifestyle change yielded a significantly lower incidence of abnormal waist circumference, hypertriglyceridemia, elevated fasting plasma glucose (FPG), and BP. In those with MetS at baseline, lifestyle change resulted in a significantly lower prevalence of each of these components at 3 years.[24]

The DPP was subsequently extended 7 years to become the DPP Outcomes Study (DPPOS), showing additional benefit in preventing T2DM in the lifestyle and metformin groups (**Table 3**).[25]

A 2011 systematic review, evaluating 58 trials of interventions for adult obesity, confirmed the DPP results, showing that behavioral interventions involving 12 to 26 sessions over a year were associated with a statistically significant 4-kg to 6.8-kg weight loss in adults. A greater number of intervention sessions were associated

Table 2
Diabetes Prevention Program

Key Findings	Lifestyle Change	Metformin	Placebo
Intervention adherence	Weight loss goal: 50% of patients achieved, 38% maintained. Exercise goal: 74% achieved, 58% maintained	72% took 80% of medication	77% took 80% of medication
Average weight loss	5.6 kg ($P<.001$)	2.1 kg	0.1 kg
T2DM incidence per 100 person-years	4.8	7.8	11.0
Cumulative T2DM incidence	14%	22%	29%
T2DM risk reduction	58%	39%	—
Number needed to treat to prevent 1 case of T2DM over 3 y	6.9	13.9	—

with more weight loss. Higher-intensity interventions involved self-monitoring, goal setting, addressing barriers to change, and developing long-term maintenance strategies. Although weight loss was modest, T2DM incidence was reduced by 50% over 2 years to 3 years. Trials had sparse outcomes data, were underpowered to address other outcomes, and did not demonstrate an effect on mortality, CVD, hospitalizations, or depression. The investigators noted that intensive behavioral interventions might be difficult for primary care practices to implement.[26] Based on these data, the United States Preventive Services Task Force (USPSTF) has provided a grade B recommendation that individuals over 18 years with a BMI greater than or equal to 30 kg/m^2 be offered or referred to intensive, multicomponent behavioral interventions, promoting a healthy diet and physical activity with the goal of reducing CVD risk.[27]

Table 3
Diabetes Prevention Program Outcomes Study key findings

	Lifestyle Change	Metformin	Placebo
Adherence to bridge intervention: some attendance at 16 group sessions	40%	58%	57%
Adherence to intervention: quarterly lifestyle sessions (Healthy Lifestyle Program)	18%	15%	14%
Adherence to intervention: 2 × 4 weekly BOOST sessions/y	17%	Not given	Not given
Weight loss	DPP initial loss 7 kg, gradual regain, maintained 2 kg net loss	Maintained original 2.5 kg loss	<1 kg loss since entry
DPP T2DM incidence per 100 person-years	4.8	7.8	11
DPPOS T2DM incidence per 100 person-years	5.9	4.9	5.6
Cumulative T2DM incidence	5.3	6.4	7.8
T2DM risk reduction since DPP randomization	34%	18%	—
Number of years T2DM delayed	4	2	—

Modeled on the DPP, the Centers for Disease Control has developed a national DPP curriculum targeting individuals at risk for T2DM. This is a structured program—in person or online—with trained coaches leading the intensive and multifaceted behavior interventions. Patients must commit to a year of weekly meetings for the first 6 months and twice-monthly meetings for another 6 months.[28] Program cost and insurance coverage vary by region. Under the Affordable Care Act, individuals obtaining health insurance through the exchanges have coverage for all preventive services recommendations graded A or B by the USPSTF, including obesity screening and counseling. There are also incentives for state coverage of USPSTF recommended services for Medicaid beneficiaries, including obesity treatment.[29]

Key resource for clinicians and patients:

DPP details can be found at: https://www.cdc.gov/diabetes/prevention/index.html.

Commercial Weight Loss Programs

A 2015 systematic review of commercial weight loss interventions compared with control/education showed some benefits from participation in commercial programs. Participants in several programs achieved greater weight loss at 12 months. Referring patients to such programs might be particularly reasonable when clinicians and practices lack time, training, or ancillary staff to provide adequate behavioral counseling.[29]

Exercise

Exercise is a cornerstone of lifestyle change and mitigates MetS through various mechanisms. There is a strong inverse association between physical activity and all-cause mortality at all levels of BMI. The greatest reduction in all-cause mortality occurs when sedentary individuals engage in even a minimal amount of daily physical activity (20 min brisk walking daily). Higher activity levels are associated with further risk reductions.[30] Recommended minimum exercise standards advise that children should engage in 60 min/d of moderate to vigorous aerobic activity. Adults should strive for 150 minutes/week of moderate intensity aerobic activity (eg, walking $\geq$4.8 km/hour or gardening) in addition to muscle-strengthening activity (working all major muscle groups) 2 d/wk. Pregnant/postpartum women should aim for 150 min/wk moderate-intensity aerobic activity. In all cases, 10-min duration intervals of activity contribute to total time.[31]

Walking is often the simplest and easiest form of physical activity available. The average US adult takes 5900 steps/d to 6900 steps/d. Daily step goals should include at least 3000 to 4000 additional steps (approximately 30 minutes total/day) for 5 d/wk in at least 10-minute intervals. Although greater than or equal to 12,500 steps/d are associated with improved cardiovascular fitness, incremental improvement in activity level is a practical, if modest, approach to encouraging exercise in inactive individuals with MetS.[32] In the context of MetS, physical activity contributes to weight loss, diastolic BP (DBP) reduction (2 mm Hg), and improvement in TG (−0.2 mmol/L) and fasting glucose (−0.2 mmol/L). Fasting glucose reductions were greater with more intense activity (−0.3 mmol/L).[33] Metabolic benefits of physical activity are independent of cardiovascular physiology changes or actual changes in weight.[34]

Sedentary behavior has emerged as a significant contributor to MetS. The average American adult sits 6 hours to 8 hours daily. Insulin sensitivity decreases with physical inactivity. Physical inactivity results in elevated postprandial glucose concentration after just 3 days. With sustained inactivity, insulin resistance increases further. Conversely, insulin sensitivity improves if periods of inactivity are interspersed with regular episodes of light or moderate activity.[35]

Dietary Approaches

Dietary Approaches to Stop Hypertension diet

BP decreases as dietary sodium decreases. The challenge to achieving a low-sodium diet is that sodium in processed foods accounts for a majority of average daily salt intake.[36] Therefore, dietary patterns, as opposed to individual nutrients, may have the most important impact on BP and MetS. In hypertensive patients adhering to the patterns outlined in the Dietary Approaches to Stop Hypertension (DASH) diet (more protein, nuts, legumes, and fish and fewer sweets or snacks), reductions in systolic BP (SBP) and diastolic BP (DBP) were equivalent to those achieved with antihypertensive drug monotherapy (**Table 4**).[37]

Mediterranean diet

The Mediterranean diet (MD) (**Table 5**) mirrors the traditional diet of olive-growing regions surrounding the Mediterranean. It is associated with a decrease in MetS and an improvement in waist circumference, FPG, TG, SBP, and HDL. Decreases in CVD, T2DM (in participants initially without T2DM), peripheral arterial disease, atrial fibrillation hypertension, and subclinical atherosclerosis have been associated with the MD as well (**Table 6**). The MD is high in unsaturated fat from natural vegetable sources and preferred over a low-fat diet for cardiovascular health, perhaps due to antioxidant and antiinflammatory effects.[38,39]

Dietary sugar

Between 1970 and 2005, American daily energy intake increased by 150 cal to 300 cal. US children 2 years to 19 years of age now consume 80 g of added sugar daily. A net energy input of 50 cal/d results in a (2.3-kg) weight gain over 1 year. Diets high in simple sugars are associated with increased inflammation and oxidative stress. In addition, diets high in sugar and fat may activate central pathways for craving. Chronic hyperinsulinemia, a result of hyperglycemia, may inhibit dopamine clearance from the nucleus accumbens, fostering food-derived pleasure and promoting excess energy intake. Added sugars consumed in either foods or beverages are associated with weight gain.[40,41]

Included in added sugars are all sugars used as ingredients in processed and prepared foods (commonly sucrose and high-fructose corn syrup, both containing fructose and glucose monosaccharides) and sugar added at the table. Other metabolic equivalents include brown sugar, corn sweetener, corn syrup, fruit juice concentrates, high-fructose corn syrup, honey, malt sugar, molasses, raw sugar, dextrose, fructose, glucose, lactose, maltose, and sucrose.[42] **Table 7** lists American Heart Association recommended daily sugar limits. As an example, a 12-oz carbonated cola beverage

Table 4 Dietary Approaches to Stop Hypertension effect on systolic blood pressure and diastolic blood pressure			
All values = mm Hg	Control	High Fruits and Vegetables	Combination Diet
Overall BP decrease	—	SBP by 2.8, DBP by 1.1	SBP by 5.5, DBP by 3.0
If hypertension, BP effect	—	—	SBP by 11, DBP by 6
If normotensive, BP effect	—	—	SBP by 3.5, DBP by 2.1

Table 5 Mediterranean diet components		
High Intake	**Moderate Intake**	**Low Intake**
Olive oil as main dietary fat	Wine (especially red wine), usually with meals	Sweets and desserts
Plant-derived foods (fruit, vegetables, legumes, nuts, seeds, and whole-grain cereals)	Dairy products (especially yogurt and cheese but not whole milk, butter, or cream)	Red and processed meats
	Seafood	
	Poultry and eggs	

contains 8 tsp or 34 g and 130 cal added sugar, approaching or exceeding daily recommended limits for added sugars.[40,41] Current food label guidelines mandate reporting of total and added sugars.[43]

Low glycemic diet

The glycemic index (GI) stratifies foods on a scale of 0 to 100 according to impact on blood sugar levels. Lower GI foods are associated improved glucose homeostasis. Low GI diets result in modest reductions in weight gain and BMI, decreases in total and LDL cholesterol, and no differences in BP. Benefits were greater in obese patients. Studies of low GI diets suggest that the type of food consumed is more important than the quantity of food consumed.[44]

Regardless of the specific diet chosen, patients with MetS should consume fewer processed and sugar-rich foods and more vegetables, fruits, and plant-based fats.

When Are Medications an Option?

In cases where lifestyle change has been inadequate, weight loss medication may facilitate achievement of weight loss goals. **Table 8** summarizes mechanism of action, efficacy, and side effects of drugs currently approved for weight loss. Trials of these medications are heterogeneous, often include components of nutritional counseling, and describe high attrition and side-effect rates. No trials have examined sustained weight loss greater than 1 year to 2 years or weight maintenance after drug discontinuation. Comorbidities, cost, tolerability, and individual preferences are important considerations when choosing a medication specifically for weight loss in patients with

Table 6 Predimed key findings			
Key Findings	**Mediterranean Diet + Olive Oil**	**Mediterranean Diet + Nuts**	**Control**
CVD rate/1000 person-years	8.1	8.0	11.2
Unadjusted hazard ratios	0.70 (CI, 0.53–0.91)	0.70 (CI, 0.53–0.94)	—
Primary CVD endpoint	ARR 1.34% NNT 75	ARR 1.25% NNT 80	—
Regression of MetS hazard ratio	1.35 (favoring regression)	1.28 (favoring regression)	—
T2DM incidence	ARR 3.52% NNT 28	ARR 1.59% (−0.88%– 3.44%)	—

Abbreviations: ARR, absolute risk reduction; NNT, number needed to treat.

Table 7		
American Heart Association daily added sugar limit		
Adult Woman	**Adult Man**	**Child**
6 tsp or	9 tsp or	6 tsp or
25 g or	36 g or	25 g or
80 cal	144 cal	100 cal
Expected energy expenditure of 1800 cal	Assumed daily energy expenditure of 2200 cal	Avoid added sugars in children <2 y of age 1 or fewer 8-oz SSBs/wk

MetS.[23,45–47] An intensive behavioral intervention has been shown to augment weight loss in combination with pharmacotherapy, further emphasizing the need for a systems based, multifaceted approach to obesity and MetS.[26]

Who Is a Candidate for Surgery?

Bariatric surgery is associated with dramatic and sustained weight loss for many patients (**Table 9**). In 1991, the National Institutes of Health published bariatric surgery guidelines considering surgery in patients with BMI greater than or equal to 40 kg/m^2 or BMI greater than or equal to 5 kg/m^2 with high-risk comorbidities (T2DM, OSA, and obesity-related cardiomyopathy). Recommendations since have trended to a lower surgery threshold.

The American Diabetes Association (ADA) recommends considering surgery for patients with a BMI greater than 35 kg/m^2 if T2DM or other comorbidities are inadequately controlled with lifestyle and pharmacologic therapy. The National Institute for Health and Care Excellence (NICE) guidelines recommends considering surgery for patients with BMI 30 kg/m^2 to 35 kg/m^2 who have a recent T2DM diagnosis.[48,49]

Surgery is associated with long-term weight loss, remission of T2DM, and significant MetS resolution compared with nonsurgical treatment at 2 years of follow-up.[49,50] Bariatric surgery has led to improvement in hypertension, hyperlipidemia, 10-year cardiovascular risk, and inflammatory markers; regression of left ventricular hypertrophy; and modest reductions in cardiovascular mortality.[51]

Although surgery is an important tool in the treatment of MetS, there are potential harms. Potential risks include reoperation for hemorrhage (2%), anastomotic leak (2%), anastomotic ulcer (8%), intestinal obstruction (5%), anastomotic stricture (5%), and death (0.03%). Bariatric surgery forces an immediate and dramatic change in lifestyle and dietary habits. As such, surgery may help stimulate significant behavioral change. Whether surgery or a comprehensive medical approach, long-term success in treating MetS requires an intense commitment.[51]

Self-Management Strategies

Online, computer-based interventions are widely used to assist with weight loss (**Table 10**).[52–58] They are moderately effective and may appeal, in particular, to younger, technology-savvy patients or help support patients enrolled in intensive behavioral interventions.[59]

CASE DISCUSSIONS REVISITED

Individual care plans should be developed with consideration of composite risk, which is facilitated by considering a patient's phenotypic subtype and stage. Treatment plans may then be developed across the continuum of care. **Fig. 3** depicts an

Table 8
Comparison of weight loss drugs

Drug	Mechanism of Action	Efficacy in Weight Loss	Comments
Orlistat (Xenical and Alli), 60–120 mg, TID	Inhibits pancreatic lipases and intestinal fat absorption	• 2.9 kg weight loss • 2.9% more weight loss vs placebo • 21% more in orlistat vs placebo achieved 5% weight loss and 12% more achieved 10% weight loss • Similar weight regain for orlistat vs placebo during weight maintenance	Additional benefits: decreased total cholesterol and LDL-cholesterol; decreased SBP of 1.5 mm Hg and DBP of 1.4 mm Hg; T2DM incidence decreased from 9.0% to 6.2%, mostly in patients with baseline glucose intolerance Side effects: 80% incidence of gastrointestinal side effects: steatorrhea, bloating, oily discharge, fecal incontinence, malabsorption of fat-soluble vitamins
Lorcaserin (Belviq), 10 mg, BID; schedule IV	Serotonin (5-HT) 2C receptor agonist to hypothalamic anorexigenic neurons; thought to inhibit appetite, promote satiety	• BMI decreased 5.8% with lorcaserin vs 2.2% with placebo • 44.1% of lorcaserin vs 20.5% placebo patients achieved 5% weight loss • 20.5% lorcaserin vs 7.3% placebo attained ≥10% loss	Common side effects: headache, nausea, and upper respiratory tract infections Serotonin syndrome risk if combined with drugs affecting serotonin clearance Other serotonergic effects: priapism, suicidal ideation, euphoria
Liraglutide (Saxenda), 0.6 mg, titrated to 3 mg SQ daily	Hypothalamic glucagon-like peptide 1 receptor agonist: regulates appetite. Direct gastrointestinal effect: vagal tone and delayed gastric emptying causing early satiety	• BMI reduction from baseline over 1 y: 6.5% liraglutide vs 1.6% in placebo • 56% of liraglutide treatment vs 23.4% placebo attained 5% weight loss • 28% liraglutide vs 7.9% placebo achieved 10% weight loss	Side effects: nausea, diarrhea, and constipation Serious adverse events (hepatobiliary, gallbladder) 6.3% in treatment group, 4.6% (infection) placebo

(continued on next page)

Table 8
(continued)

Drug	Mechanism of Action	Efficacy in Weight Loss	Comments
Rimonabant, 20 mg daily (European approval for long-term use)	Endocannabinoid system inhibitor: central and peripheral mechanisms to reduce food intake	• 4.7 kg more weight loss for rimonabant vs placebo Rimonabant vs placebo increased 5% weight loss by 33% and 10% loss by 19%	Caution: increased incidence of psychiatric disorders Contraindicated for patients with severe depression and not recommended for patients with untreated psychiatric conditions
Metformin (off-label use for weight loss), 850 mg, daily to BID	Biguanide antihyperglycemic	• DPP average weight loss was 0.1 kg, 2.1 kg, and 5.6 kg in the placebo, metformin, and lifestyle groups ($P<.001$)	Additional benefits: metformin reduced the prevalence of low HDL, increased waist circumference, and elevated FPG Side effects: gastrointestinal symptoms
Phentermine/topiramate extended release (Qsymia) 3.75/23–15/92 mg, daily; schedule IV	Phentermine: sympathomimetic amine anorectic; may cause hypothalamic catecholamine release, suppressing appetite Topiramate: neurostabilizer with unclear mechanism for weight loss: possible appetite suppression and increased satiety Additive effect	• Dose-related BMI reduction 5.1%–10.9% • At maximum dose: 66.7%–70.0% of patients achieved 5% weight loss and 47.2%–48.0% attained 10% weight loss • Sustained weight reductions in 1 y continuation study	Additional benefits: dose-dependent improvements over placebo in SBP, DBP, LDL, HDL, and TG Side effects: dose-dependent paresthesias, constipation, dry mouth. Increased resting heart rate. May have increased risk depression, anxiety, and irritability; caution if concurrent mood disorder
Naltrexone/bupropion, 16/180 mg, BID	Bupropion: dopamine and norepinephrine reuptake inhibitor Naltrexone: opioid receptor antagonist Hypothalamic melanocortin and mesolimbic reward system activity, affecting food intake regulation	• BMI reduction of 6.7% with naltrexone/bupropion vs 2.4% with placebo • With naltrexone/bupropion, 52.4% of patients attained 5% weight loss and 28.3% of patients attained 10% vs 23.6% and 9.7% with placebo	Side effects: nausea, constipation, and headache Caution: bupropion: black box warning for increased risk of pediatric suicidality; neuropsychiatric reactions

Table 9 Bariatric surgery excess weight lost over time			
Procedure	1 Year	3–10 Years	10 or More Years
Roux-en-Y gastric bypass	62%	50%–60%	54%
Laparoscopic adjustable gastric band	48%	50%–60%	54%
Vertical banded gastroplasty	68%	—	—
Biliopancreatic diversion procedure	70%	70%	72%

integrative model of care that encourages investment by all potential stakeholders to contribute to both individual and community patient identification and treatment approaches.

Case 1: Metabolic Syndrome Phenotype: Adiposity, Vascular, Other; Stage D

Clinically this patient has multiple parameters that may fall below usual treatment thresholds; however, his MetS risk assessment is high. Disease-specific therapies include treatment of gout with urate-lowering therapy; evaluating hepatic steatosis; aggressive lifestyle assessment, including BP monitoring; and evaluation for end-organ disease, including OSA and T2DM. Additional considerations include referral to a DPP program and, depending on his progress over time, weight loss pharmaco-therapy or bariatric surgery.

Case 2: Metabolic Syndrome Phenotype: Insulin Resistance, Other; Stage B

This patient should focus on weight loss with a goal of reversing insulin resistance and normalizing menses to optimize fertility. Specific measures could include referral to nutrition or commercial weight loss program or the DPP, advice to exercise at least 30 minutes 5 d/wk, and a metformin prescription.

Case 3: Metabolic Syndrome Phenotype: Lipid Dominant, Insulin Resistance; Stage C

It is essential that she initiate therapy with aggressive lifestyle modification focusing on weight loss and lipid management. Her long-term wellness requires addressing her diet and activity habits. Motivational interviewing would identify her barriers to change and learning style and facilitate adapting modalities to fit her needs. This might include the use of educational and self-management Web resources in addition to or in place of conventional or commercial lifestyle change strategies. If sedentary, she could achieve substantial benefit by adopting a modest incremental increase in activity of 20 minutes of brisk walking daily. Her treatment should include lipid management with careful consideration for the use of a statin in this reproductive-age woman. Assessment must include evaluation of her sugar intake, especially her use of SSBs. Daily sugar intake should be limited to no more than 24 g to 25 g (5–6 tsp). In-office nutrition counseling could emphasize the MD or GI diet.

Case 4: Metabolic Syndrome Phenotype: Preadiposity Dominant, Pre-insulin Resistance; Stage A

Simply performing a Papanicolaou smear and failing to recognize and address her emerging MetS would underserve this patient. Appropriate goals for this patient include preventing further weight gain, normalizing BMI, and increasing activity to pre-vent MetS progression. She should be screened for other criteria for MetS and pro-vided specific lifestyle advice, including an exercise prescription beginning with a recommendation to get up and move every 20 minutes for at least 2 minutes. She

Table 10
Web resources for diet and fitness

Organization	Web Site	Site Features
American Heart Association	www.heart.org	Discusses obesity-related disease on individual and population level and across the life span. Multifaceted recommendations: weight loss, healthy eating, reducing sedentary behavior, increasing activity Does not endorse any single diet (DASH mentioned, recommendations aligned with MD) Recommends water instead of SSBs Detailed and graphic resources
Dr Weil, advocates for integrative medicine	www.drweil.com	Emphasizes healthy living, exercise, and antiinflammatory diet Antiinflammatory diet: vegetables, fruit, beans, legumes, grains, nuts, Asian mushrooms, herbs, spices, healthy sweets Emphasis on supplements and alternative food pyramid Recipes include some obscure ingredients Best for audience interested in alternative medicine
US Department of Agriculture	www.nutrition.gov	Targets health and policy professionals Healthy People 2015–2120 executive summary Variety of nutrition topics: general, vegetarian, diabetes (including gestational), allergy/food sensitivity, disordered eating
US Department of Agriculture	www.choosemyplate.gov	English/Spanish Variety of diet topics Table with synonyms for added sugars Discusses different fats/sodium Recommends limiting sweets, but menus include sweets, juices
MyFitnessPal (owned by athletic apparel company Under Armour)	MyFitnessPal.com	Food and activity tracking—numbers and calorie oriented Online and mobile app community Weight loss stories Basic program free, premium an option
US Department of Agriculture	www.supertracker.usda.gov	Based on MyPlate Interactive: nutrition data by food, serving, or meal Visual and graph data regarding daily goals Tracks activity, monitors goals
Produce for Better Health Foundation (nonprofit) partnered with Centers for Disease Control	www.fruitsandveggiesmorematters.org	Focus on fruit and vegetables Visual teaching: meal makeovers Recipe videos

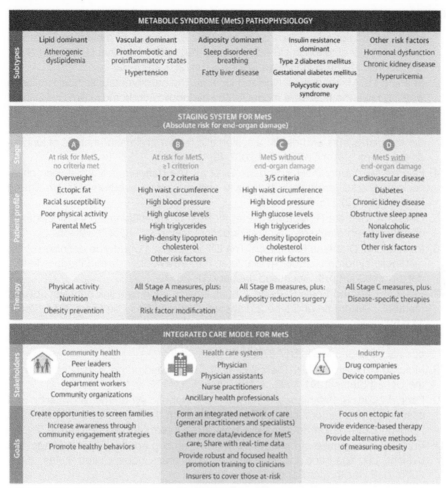

METABOLIC SYNDROME (MetS) PATHOPHYSIOLOGY				
Lipid dominant	**Vascular dominant**	**Adiposity dominant**	**Insulin resistance dominant**	**Other risk factors**
Atherogenic dyslipidemia	Prothrombotic and proinflammatory states	Sleep disordered breathing	Type 2 diabetes mellitus	Hormonal dysfunction
	Hypertension	Fatty liver disease	Gestational diabetes mellitus	Chronic kidney disease
			Polycystic ovary syndrome	Hyperuricemia

STAGING SYSTEM FOR MetS (Absolute risk for end-organ damage)			
A	**B**	**C**	**D**
At risk for MetS, no criteria met	At risk for MetS, ≥1 criterion	MetS without end-organ damage	MetS with end-organ damage
Overweight	1 or 2 criteria	3/5 criteria	Cardiovascular disease
Ectopic fat	High waist circumference	High waist circumference	Diabetes
Racial susceptibility	High blood pressure	High blood pressure	Chronic kidney disease
Poor physical activity	High glucose levels	High glucose levels	Obstructive sleep apnea
Parental MetS	High triglycerides	High triglycerides	Nonalcoholic fatty liver disease
	High-density lipoprotein cholesterol	High-density lipoprotein cholesterol	Other risk factors
	Other risk factors	Other risk factors	
Physical activity	All Stage A measures, plus:	All Stage B measures, plus:	All Stage C measures, plus:
Nutrition	Medical therapy	Adiposity reduction surgery	Disease-specific therapies
Obesity prevention	Risk factor modification		

INTEGRATED CARE MODEL FOR MetS		
Community health	Health care system	Industry
Peer leaders	Physician	Drug companies
Community health department workers	Physician assistants	Device companies
Community organizations	Nurse practitioners	
	Ancillary health professionals	
Create opportunities to screen families	Form an integrated network of care (general practitioners and specialists)	Focus on ectopic fat
Increase awareness through community engagement strategies	Gather more data/evidence for MetS care; Share with real-time data	Provide evidence-based therapy
Promote healthy behaviors	Provide robust and focused health promotion training to clinicians	Provide alternative methods of measuring obesity
	Insurers to cover those at-risk	

Fig. 3. MetS: integrated care for patients. (*From* Sperling LS, Mechanick JI, Neeland IJ, et al. The cardiometabolic health alliance working toward a new care model for the metabolic syndrome. J Am Coll Cardiol 2015;66(9):1050–67; with permission.)

should aspire to increase her regular activity. Because walking is easily initiated, she could be advised to include 150 min/wk. This could also be achieved by adding an additional 3000 to 4000 steps/d 5 d/wk in at least 10-minute intervals.

SUMMARY

MetS is common in primary care. Consideration of the phenotypic presentations, applying the defining criteria, and appropriately staging these patients allow clinicians to consistently identify and treat MetS patients before prothrombotic and proinflammatory processes alter end-organ function. Treatment centers on changes in dietary and physical activity patterns. Success often requires systems thinking and implementation of a multidisciplinary team. Medications and surgery are other options available to achieve weight loss essential to preventing and treating morbidity and mortality associated with MetS.

REFERENCES

1. Miller JM, Kaylor MB, Johannsson M, et al. Prevalence of metabolic syndrome and individual criterion in US adolescents: 2001-2010 National Health and Nutrition Survey. Metab Syndr Relat Disord 2014;12(10):527–32.
2. Sperling LS, Mechanick JI, Neeland IJ, et al. The cardiometabolic health alliance working toward a new care model for the metabolic syndrome. J Am Coll Cardiol 2015;66(9):1050–67.
3. Gami AS, Witt BJ, Howard DE, et al. Metabolic syndrome and risk of incident cardiovascular events and death: a systematic review and meta-analysis of longitudinal studies. J Am Coll Cardiol 2007;49(4):403–14.
4. Faienza MF, Wang DQH, Fruhbeck G, et al. The dangerous link between childhood and adult predictors of obesity and metabolic syndrome. Intern Emerg Med 2016;11(2):175–82.
5. Ohashi K, Shibata R, Murohara T, et al. Role of anti-inflammatory adipokines in obesity-related diseases. Trends Endocrinol Metab 2014;25(7):348–55.
6. International Diabetes Federation. The IDF consensus worldwide definition of the metabolic syndrome, 2006. Available at: http://www.idf.org/webdata/docs/MetS_def_update2006.pdf. Accessed January 31, 2017.
7. Esser N, Legrand-Poels S, Piette J, et al. Inflammation as a link between obesity, metabolic syndrome and type 2 diabetes. Diabetes Res Clin Pract 2014;105(2):141–50.
8. Heymsfield SB, Wadden TA. Mechanisms, pathophysiology, and management of obesity. N Engl J Med 2017;376(3):254–66.
9. Mokdad AH, Serdula MK, Dietz WH, et al. The spread of the obesity epidemic in the United States 1991-1998. JAMA 1999;282(16):1519–22.
10. Park YW, Zhu S, Palaniappan L, et al. The metabolic syndrome: prevalence and associated risk factors in the US population from the Third National Health and Nutrition Examination Survey 1988-1994. Arch Intern Med 2003;163(4):427–36.
11. Ervin RB. Prevalence of metabolic syndrome among adults 20 years of age and over, by sex, age, race and ethnicity, and body mass index: United States, 2003-2006. Natl Health Stat Report 2009;(13):1–7.
12. Karpe F, Dickmann JR, Frayn KN. Fatty acids, obesity and insulin resistance: time for a reevaluation. Diabetes 2011;60(10):2441–9.
13. Kondo K, Shibata R, Unno K, et al. Impact of a single intracoronary administration of adiponectin on myocardial ischemia/reperfusion injury in a pig model. Circ Cardiovasc Interv 2010;3(2):166–73.
14. Tune JD, Goodwill AG, Sassoon DJ, et al. Cardiovascular consequences of metabolic syndrome. Transl Res 2017. https://doi.org/10.1016/j.trsl.2017.01.001.
15. Via MA, Mechanick JI. Nutrition in type 2 diabetes and the metabolic syndrome. Med Clin North Am 2016;100(6):1285–302. Available at: https://doi.org/10.1016/j.mcna.2016.06.009.
16. Koster A, Stenholm S, Alley DE, et al. Body fat distribution and inflammation among obese older adults with and without metabolic syndrome. Obesity (Silver Spring) 2010;18(12):2354–61.
17. Bozkurt B, Aguilar D, Deswal A, et al. Contributory risk and management of comorbidities of hypertension, obesity, diabetes mellitus, hyperlipidemia and metabolic syndrome in chronic heart failure: a scientific statement from the American Heart Association. Circulation 2016;134(23):e535–78.
18. Lustig RH. Fructose: it's "alcohol without the buzz". Adv Nutr 2013;4(2):226–35.

19. Stanhope KL. Sugar consumption, metabolic disease and obesity: the state of the controversy. Crit Rev Clin Lab Sci 2016;53(1):52–67.
20. Kanbay M, Jensen T, Solak Y, et al. Uric acid in metabolic syndrome: from an innocent bystander to a central player. Eur J Intern Med 2016;29:3–8.
21. Beattie CJ, Fulton RL, Higgins P, et al. Allopurinol initiation and change in blood pressure in older adults with hypertension. Hypertension 2014;64(5):1102–7.
22. Girman CJ, Dekker JM, Rhodes T, et al. An exploratory analysis of criteria for the metabolic syndrome and its prediction of long-term cardiovascular outcomes: the Hoorn study. Am J Epidemiol 2005;162(5):438–47.
23. Diabetes Prevention Program Research Group. Reduction in the incidence of type 2 diabetes with lifestyle intervention or metformin. N Engl J Med 2002; 346(6):393–403. Available at: http://www.nejm.org.offcampus.lib.washington. edu/doi/full/10.1056/NEJMoa012512.
24. Orchard TJ, Temprosa M, Goldberg R, et al. The effect of metformin and intensive lifestyle intervention on the metabolic syndrome: the diabetes prevention program. Ann Intern Med 2005;142(8):611–9. Available at: https://www-ncbi-nlm-nih-gov.offcampus.lib.washington.edu/pmc/articles/PMC2505046/.
25. Diabetes Prevention Program Research Group. 10-year follow-up of diabetes incidence and weight loss in the diabetes prevention program outcomes study. Lancet 2009;374:1677–86. Available at: https://www-ncbi-nlm-nih-gov. offcampus.lib.washington.edu/pmc/articles/PMC3135022/.
26. LeBlanc E, O'Connor E, Whitlock E, et al. Review annals of internal medicine effectiveness of primary care – relevant treatments for obesity. Ann Intern Med 2011;155:434–47. Available at: https://www-ncbi-nlm-nih-gov.offcampus.lib. washington.edu/pubmedhealth/PMH0031764/.
27. Moyer VA. Screening for and management of obesity in adults: U.S. Preventive services task force recommendation statement. Ann Intern Med 2012;157(5):373–8. Available at: http://annals.org.offcampus.lib.washington.edu/aim/article/1355696/ screening-management-obesity-adults-u-s-preventive-services-task-force.
28. Available at: https://www.cdc.gov/diabetes/prevention/index.html. Accessed February 28, 2017.
29. Gudzune KA, Doshi RS, Mehta AK, et al. Efficacy of commercial weight loss programs: an updated systematic review. Ann Intern Med 2015;162(7):501–12. Efficacy. Available at: https://www.ncbi.nlm.nih.gov/pmc/articles/PMC4446719/.
30. Ekelund U, Ward H a, Norat T, et al. Physical activity and all-cause mortality across levels of overall and abdominal adiposity in European men and women: the European Prospective Investigation into Cancer and Nutrition Study (EPIC). 1 – 6 The EPIC cohort. Am J Clin Nutr 2015;101(3):613–21. Available at: http:// ajcn.nutrition.org.offcampus.lib.washington.edu/content/101/3/613.full.pdf+html.
31. Available at: https://www.cdc.gov/physicalactivity/basics/index.htm. Accessed March 15, 2017.
32. Tudor-Locke C. Steps to better cardiovascular health: how many steps does it take to achieve good health and how confident are we in this number? Curr Cardiovasc Risk Rep 2010;4:271–6. Available at: https://www-ncbi-nlm-nih-gov.offcampus.lib. washington.edu/pmc/articles/PMC2894114/pdf/12170_2010_Article_109.pdf.
33. Shaw K, Gennat H, O'Rourke P, et al. Exercise for overweight or obesity. Cochrane Database Syst Rev 2006. https://doi.org/10.1002/14651858.CD003817. pub3. Available at: http://onlinelibrary.wiley.com.offcampus.lib.washington.edu/ doi/10.1002/14651858.CD003817.pub3/epdf/abstract.
34. Pandey A, Swift D, McGuire D, et al. Metabolic effects of exercise training among fitness nonresponsive patients with type 2 diabetes: the HART-D study.

Diabetes Care 2015;38:1494–501. Available at: http://care.diabetesjournals.org.
offcampus.lib.washington.edu/content/38/8/1494.long.

35. Young DR, Hivert M-F, Alhassan S, et al. Sedentary behavior and cardiovascular
morbidity and mortality: a science advisory from the American Heart Association.
Circulation 2016;134. https://doi.org/10.1161/CIR.0000000000000440. Available
at: http://circ.ahajournals.org.offcampus.lib.washington.edu/content/134/13/e262.
long.

36. Sacks F, Svetkey L, Vollmer W, et al. Effects on blood pressure of reduced dietary
sodium and the dietary approaches to stop hypertension (DASH) diet. N Engl J
Med 2001;344(1):3–10. Available at: https://www-ncbi-nlm-nih-gov.offcampus.lib.
washington.edu/pubmed/1113695.

37. Appel L, Moore T, Obarzanek E, et al. A clinical trial of the effects of dietary patterns on
blood pressure. N Engl J Med 1997;336(16):1117–24. Available at: http://www.nejm.
org.offcampus.lib.washington.edu/doi/pdf/10.1056/NEJM199704173361601.

38. Martínez-González MA, Salas-Salvadó J, Estruch R, et al. Benefits of the mediterranean diet: insights from the PREDIMED study. Prog Cardiovasc Dis 2015;58(1):
50–60. Available at: http://www.sciencedirect.com.offcampus.lib.washington.
edu/science/article/pii/S0033062015000286.

39. Kastorini CM, Milionis HJ, Esposito K, et al. The effect of mediterranean diet on metabolic syndrome and its components: a meta-analysis of 50 studies and 534,906 individuals. J Am Coll Cardiol 2011;57:1299–313. Available at: http://www.sciencedirect.
com.offcampus.lib.washington.edu/science/article/pii/S0735109710050679. Accessed January 31, 2017.

40. Johnson RK, Appel LJ, Brands M, et al. Dietary sugars intake and cardiovascular
health a scientific statement from the american heart association. Circulation
2009;120(11):1011–20. Available at: http://circ.ahajournals.org.offcampus.lib.
washington.edu/content/120/11/1011.long.

41. Vos MB, Kaar JL, Welsh JA, et al. Added sugars and cardiovascular disease risk
in children: a scientific statement from the American Heart Association. Circulation
2016. https://doi.org/10.1161/CIR.0000000000000439. http://circ.ahajournals.org.
offcampus.lib.washington.edu/content/early/2016/08/22/CIR.0000000000000439.
long.

42. Available at: http://www.heart.org/HEARTORG/HealthyLiving/HealthyEating/
Nutrition/Sugar-101_UCM_306024_Article.jsp#3_finding_added_sugars_in_food.
Accessed January 13, 2017.

43. Available at: https://www.regulations.gov/document?D=FDA-2012-N-1210-0875.
Accessed January 13, 2017.

44. Thomas DE, Elliott EJ, Baur L. Low glycaemic index or low glycaemic load diets
for overweight and obesity [review]. Cochrane Database Syst Rev 2007;(3).
CD005105. Available at: http://onlinelibrary.wiley.com.offcampus.lib.washington.
edu/doi/10.1002/14651858.CD005105.pub2/epdf/abstract.

45. Padwal R, Li SK, Lau DC. Long-term pharmacotherapy for obesity and overweight
[review]. Cochrane Database Syst Rev 2004;(3). CD004094. Available at: http://
onlinelibrary.wiley.com.offcampus.lib.washington.edu/doi/10.1002/14651858.
CD004094.pub2/abstract. Accessed January 31, 2017.

46. Emili A, Abushomar H, Nair K. Treating metabolic syndrome: lifestyle change or
medication? Can Fam Physician 2007;53(7):1203–5. Available at: http://www.
cfp.ca.offcampus.lib.washington.edu/content/53/7/1203.long.

47. Nuffer W, Trujillo JM, Megyeri J. A comparison of new pharmacological agents
for the treatment of obesity. Ann Pharmacother 2016;50(5):376–88. Available
at: http://journals.sagepub.com.offcampus.lib.washington.edu/doi/abs/10.1177

/1060028016634351?url_ver=Z39.88-2003&rfr_id=ori:rid:crossref.org&rfr_dat=cr_pub%3dpubmed.

48. Genser L, Casella Mariolo JR, Castagneto-Gissey L, et al. Obesity, type 2 diabetes, and the metabolic syndrome: pathophysiologic relationships and guidelines for surgical intervention. Surg Clin North Am 2016;96(4):681–701. Available at: http://www.sciencedirect.com.offcampus.lib.washington.edu/science/article/pii/S0039610916300135.

49. O'Brien P. Surgical treatment of obesity. In: De Groot LJ, Chrousos G, Dungan K, et al, editors. Endotext. South Dartmouth (MA): MDText.com; 2016. https://www-ncbi-nlm-nih-gov.offcampus.lib.washington.edu/books/NBK279090/. Accessed January 31, 2017.

50. Colquitt JL, Pickett K, Loveman E, et al. Surgery for weight loss in adults [review]. Cochrane Database Syst Rev 2014;(8). CD003641. Available at: http://onlinelibrary.wiley.com.offcampus.lib.washington.edu/doi/10.1002/14651858.CD003641.pub4/full.

51. Vest AR, Heneghan HM, Agarwal S, et al. Bariatric surgery and cardiovascular outcomes: a systematic review. Heart 2012;98:1763–77. Available at: http://heart.bmj.com.offcampus.lib.washington.edu/content/heartjnl/98/24/1763.full.pdf.

52. Available at: www.heart.org. Accessed March 1, 2017.

53. Available at: www.drweil.com. Accessed March 1, 2017.

54. Available at: www.nutrition.gov. Accessed March 1, 2017.

55. Available at: www.choosemyplate.gov. Accessed March 1, 2017.

56. Available at: www.myfitnesspal.com. Accessed March 1, 2017.

57. Available at: www.supertracker.usda.gov. Accessed March 1, 2017.

58. Available at: www.fruitsandveggiesmorematters.org. Accessed March 1, 2017.

59. Wieland LS, Falzon L, Sciamanna CN, et al. Interactive computer-based interventions for weight loss or weight maintenance in overweight or obese people [review]. Cochrane Database Syst Rev 2012;(8). CD007675. Available at: www.cochranelibrary.com http://onlinelibrary.wiley.com.offcampus.lib.washington.edu/doi/10.1002/14651858.CD007675.pub2/epdf/abstract.

Cardiovascular Disease in Women

Elizabeth Anne Leonard, MD[a,b,*], Robert James Marshall, MD[c,d,1]

KEYWORDS

- Cardiovascular disease in women • Nonobstructive coronary artery disease
- Spontaneous coronary artery dissection • Takotsubo cardiomyopathy
- Pregnancy-related cardiac conditions • Preeclampsia and cardiovascular disease
- Cardiotoxicity of breast cancer therapy

KEY POINTS

- The clinical presentation of cardiovascular disease in women differs from that in men. These differences may be related specifically to genetic differences between men and women; anatomic and physiologic distinctions based on gender; and psychosocial, cultural, or economic differences.
- Traditional cardiovascular risk factors have a different impact in women than in men. Tobacco use, type 2 diabetes mellitus, obesity, depression, and psychosocial stress have a more potent effect on cardiovascular disease in women.
- Hormonal changes at different stages of a woman's life have an impact on the development of cardiovascular disease. These changes influence the cardiac conduction system, microvascular and endothelial function, and systemic inflammation.
- Pregnancy and breast cancer treatments have an impact on the development and presentation of cardiac disease. Other presentations predominantly affecting women include spontaneous coronary artery dissection and Takotsubo cardiomyopathy and likely reflect unique gender-based pathophysiology.
- Current cardiovascular prevention and treatment guidelines are developed from data obtained from mostly male subjects. These fail to account for sex-based differences that may alter risk, clinical presentation, evaluation, and therapy. The diagnosis, evaluation, and treatment of female patients should respect these guidelines, while considering distinct differences between the genders. New research specifically focusing on cardiovascular disease in women is imperative.

Disclosure: The authors have nothing to disclose.
[a] United States Navy, Camp Lejeune Family Medicine Residency, 100 Brewster Boulevard, Camp Lejeune, NC 28547, USA; [b] Uniformed Services University of the Health Sciences, Bethesda, MD, USA; [c] Cardiocare, LLC; [d] George Washington University Hospital, Washington, DC, USA
[1] Present address: 5052 Macomb Street Northwest, Washington, DC 20016.
* Corresponding author. United States Navy, 100 Brewster Boulevard, Camp Lejeune, NC 28547.
E-mail address: Elizabeth.a.leonard2.mil@mail.mil

EPIDEMIOLOGY OF CARDIOVASCULAR DISEASE IN WOMEN

Cardiovascular disease (CVD) affects 6.6 million women in the United States annually and is the leading source of morbidity and mortality among women.[1–3] Sadly, only 56% of women are aware of these statistics.[4,5] Among women diagnosed with cardiovascular disease, 2.7 million have a history of myocardial infarction. Each year more than 53,000 women die of a heart attack and 262,000 are hospitalized because of CVD.[4] One in 4 female patients presenting with a first myocardial infarction die within a year of diagnosis. Women under 45 have a higher mortality rate compared with men.[6] Although overall rates of CVD are declining, women continue to experience a disproportionately higher mortality rate.

It is projected that by 2030, $918 billion will be spent annually on CVD.[7] Although male and female patients often present differently, the long-term disease burden is similar. Female patients tend to present later in the disease process and with greater associated morbidity and mortality. Although women with CVD can present with some symptoms similar to those in men, there are clear distinctions. Women with CVD often present with broader range of symptoms than men. Obstructive coronary artery disease in women is identified less frequently than in men when relying exclusively on typical "anginal" symptoms. Often, these symptoms are commonly dismissed as noncardiac in female patients, inherently altering diagnosis and treatment patterns.

Because obstructive epicardial coronary artery atherosclerosis is less prominent as a disease in women, the term, *ischemic heart disease (IHD)*, better approximates the nature of coronary pathophysiology seen in the female population. IHD in women includes classic coronary atherosclerosis and includes disorders, such as coronary microvascular dysfunction, endothelial dysfunction, vasomotor abnormalities, and spontaneous coronary artery dissection (SCAD).[8] Other conditions thought not primarily due to a coronary cause but which predominantly affect women include postpartum and stress-induced cardiomyopathy. The classification of CVD in women, therefore, encompasses many forms of coronary and noncoronary pathology.[9] A greater variation of the cause of IHD and the diminished sensitivity and specificity of current cardiovascular testing techniques have all led to misdiagnosis and underdiagnosis of cardiac-based chest pain syndromes in women, contributing to a disproportionately greater cardiovascular morbidity and mortality.

CORONARY MICROVASCULAR DYSFUNCTION

In women, underlying CVD must be considered prominently in the differential diagnosis of chest pain syndromes regardless of age. IHD may involve both limited coronary flow reserve and endothelial dysfunction with or without atherosclerotic epicardial coronary disease.[10] Endothelial dysfunction is a vascular pathophysiology[11] that may be more common in states with low levels of estrogen.[4,10] Endothelial dysfunction may be the primary mechanism by which conditions, such as menopause, premature ovarian failure, and functional hypothalamic amenorrhea, are associated with a higher risk of CVD.[12,13] Endothelial dysfunction is also associated with inflammatory conditions, including autoimmune disorders, such as lupus or rheumatoid arthritis, the prevalence of which is increased in female patients.[5] Endothelial dysfunction leads to poor vasodilatory responsiveness, vascular smooth muscle proliferation, and increased lipid deposition.

Endothelial dysfunction, however, does not fully explain cardiac chest pain in the presence of patent coronary arteries, especially in younger women. Women may present with classic anginal symptoms and show objective evidence of inducible ischemia on stress testing but still have normal angiographic findings with either coronary CT angiography or cardiac catheterization. IHD in younger women may be mediated by non–endothelial-dependent microvascular dysfunction.[12] Mechanisms, such as recurrent microplaque rupture and erosion, also may lead to small vessel ischemia and subsequent clinical disease.

SPECIFIC NUANCE OF HEART DISEASE IN WOMEN: SPONTANEOUS CORONARY ARTERY DISSECTION, APICAL BALLOONING SYNDROME, CORONARY VASOSPASM, AND HEART FAILURE

SCAD, apical ballooning syndrome (Takotsubo cardiomyopathy), heart failure with preserved ejection fraction (HFpEF), and postural orthostatic tachycardia syndrome may contribute disproportionately to the burden of CVD in women.[9] Women are more susceptible to arteriolar and microvascular dysfunction as well as epicardial coronary vasospasm. This can lead to spontaneous or inducible acute or chronic ischemia without obstructive coronary disease. Microvascular dysfunction and/or epicardial vasospasm can lead to isolated or recurrent infarction and ischemic cardiomyopathy and also may play a role in triggering stress-induced cardiomyopathy. Signs, symptoms, and manifestations of CVD attributable to microvascular dysfunction and/or epicardial vasospasm are significantly greater in women. The hormonal influence on coronary pathophysiology also varies by age, emotional state, and personality type.[14]

SCAD is the separation of the layers of the coronary arterial wall leading to complete or partial vessel closure. SCAD should be suspected in young women who present with acute coronary syndrome (ACS) symptoms but without typical risk factors for atherosclerosis. The pathophysiology of coronary dissection is typically unrelated to atherosclerosis. SCAD is reported in 0.2% to 4% of all patients undergoing coronary angiography and in up to 11% of women under the age of 50 presenting with ACS or acute myocardial infarction. SCAD is more common in the peripartum and postpartum periods and is also associated with oral contraceptive use, connective tissue diseases, and vasculitides.[9,15] SCAD is responsible for 80% of myocardial infarctions during pregnancy.[9] It has a 10-year mortality rate of 8% and a 48% risk for major adverse cardiovascular events, including death, recurrent SCAD, myocardial infarction, and heart failure.[15] Contraception should be strongly recommended after a diagnosis of SCAD because of the high risk with subsequent pregnancies. SCAD can be a diagnostic challenge because it presents with typical and atypical angina symptoms in a population that does not have classic CVD risk factors.

Takotsubo cardiomyopathy (apical ballooning syndrome) is seen in 1% to 2% of patients who present with signs and symptoms of ACS. The exact pathophysiology of the syndrome is not clear. Characteristic regional left ventricular wall motion abnormalities are associated with this condition and are usually reversible. Troponin elevation and ischemic ECG changes are common, but there is typically no angiographic evidence of acute plaque rupture or occlusive coronary disease (even though atherosclerotic coronary artery disease may be identified). Furthermore, the affected ventricular territory does not usually correspond to a specific coronary distribution; 90% of the patients affected by Takotsubo cardiomyopathy are women between the ages of 61 and 76. Catecholamine excess is thought to play a role in the development of the syndrome because dyspnea and chest pain are the most common presenting symptoms, usually after an intense emotional reaction.[9,16] Microvascular and endothelial dysfunction also likely contribute.[16] Treatment of Takotsubo cardiomyopathy is similar to that of ACS. Once diagnosed, there is increased risk for recurrence. It is not clear whether long-term treatment with ß-blockers, ACE inhibitors, and/or angiotensin receptor blockers reduces future cardiovascular events, even if ventricular ejection fraction recovers fully.[17]

HFpEF is more common in women as opposed to left ventricular systolic dysfunction, which is more common in men.[18] Diastolic left ventricular dysfunction (impaired relaxation) is usually implicated in HFpEF and the prevalence is higher with advancing age, hypertension, and underlying IHD. HFpEF and heart failure and low left ventricular ejection fraction have a similar prognosis with an increased 5-year morbidity and mortality.[18] Other factors that may exacerbate diastolic left ventricular dysfunction and result in heart failure symptoms include atrial fibrillation, valvular heart disease, thyroid disease, and sleep apnea. Heart failure with low ejection fraction in women is associated with coronary disease, prior myocardial infarction, thyroid disease, cardiotoxic chemotherapy and peripartum cardiomyopathy (PPCM).[19] Brain natriuretic peptide helps diagnose heart failure but does not correlate with left ventricular ejection fraction. In women, a brain natriuretic peptide level greater than 500 is a stronger predictor of death than in men.[20]

ATHEROSCLEROTIC CORONARY OCCLUSIVE DISEASE IN WOMEN

Occlusive coronary artery disease remains an important etiology for cardiac symptoms in women.[3] Atherosclerotic coronary artery disease occurs later in women (average age of 72 years) than men (average age of 65).[4] The disease also carries a different prognosis and has a different demographic and risk factor profile compared to men. On presentation with ACS due to plaque rupture, women have an increased risk of complications, including congestive heart failure, cardiogenic shock, severe mitral regurgitation, and left ventricular free wall rupture despite presenting with a smaller infarct size overall than men.[4] Women respond to treatment differently from men, having a higher mortality rate and risk of complications after thrombolytic therapy for acute myocardial infarction, and have a higher rate of bleeding with dual antiplatelet therapy after myocardial infarction and coronary intervention.[4]

When evaluating patients, it is important to recognize that men and women have important differences in pain perception that may affect the character of symptoms in women with acute or chronic CVD.[21] Recognizing that typical cardiac symptoms occurring in a woman of any age may represent true CVD is just as important as appreciating the potential for a broad range of atypical symptoms.[22] Unfamiliarity among patients and clinicians about how CVD may present differently in women has had a negative impact on timing and intensity of therapy as well as adherence to clinical guidelines.

Women tend to present later in the disease process, often with vague symptomatology that contributes to missed and delayed diagnoses. Subtle prodromal symptoms, such as fatigue, nausea, sleep disturbance, and shortness of breath, may occur prior to or instead of more typical cardiac symptoms. The insidious nature of symptoms and differences in pain tolerance or perception, different coping mechanisms, and different cultural expectations in women likely contribute to the later to presentation to medical care and increased morbidity and mortality in women with CVD.[23] When women do present with typical anginal symptoms, however, it is more likely representative of true ACS compared with men with similar symptoms.[23] Whatever the symptoms, from tooth pain to nausea, particularly if provoked by exertion and affecting functional capability, in women the likelihood of CVD is high. Psychosocial stress also seems to increase the risk of cardiovascular events in women.[24] Despite recognized differences in how and when women present with CVD, the development of a female-specific algorithm to risk stratify patients based on symptoms remains difficult and has not been shown to improve diagnostic timeliness or accuracy.[21]

Depending on the clinical likelihood of IHD, functional cardiovascular testing is often used for risk stratification. The results of functional cardiovascular tests are less reliable in women for a variety of reasons. These include lower exercise tolerance, a difference in body shape, and the overall lack of test sensitivity or specificity in women. Nonspecific ECG changes are particularly common in women during stress testing[23] and vary with reproductive hormone levels. These have an impact on the accuracy of diagnostic testing depending on timing of the menstrual cycle or factors related to menopause and hormone replacement therapy. Clinical symptoms, functional status, and body habitus help determine which diagnostic modality is best for identifying underlying CVD.[25]

CVD risk factors vary by age and reproductive status. Prior to menopause, fewer women have hypertension, hyperlipidemia, and diabetes compared with men.[6] After menopause, the prevalence of cardiac risk factors in women approaches that of men and concurrently increases the risk of CVD later in life. Tobacco use, diabetes, depression, and other psychosocial influences are stronger predictors of cardiovascular risk in women than in men, underscoring the importance of identifying and addressing these risk factors as early as possible. Psychosocial factors and emotional stress are especially strong predictors of cardiovascular mortality in women. Inducible ischemia in response to mental stress is associated with a twofold increased risk of mortality and recurrent cardiovascular events.[26,27] Marital stress, in particular, has been implicated in the development of subsequent cardiac events.

HORMONAL DIFFERENCES: PHYSIOLOGIC AND IATROGENIC

Epidemiologic data regarding the cardiovascular effects of reproductive hormones are conflicting. Women undergo unique hormonal changes throughout their lives through primary physiologic changes, such as pregnancy and menopause, or secondarily due to disease processes, such as polycystic ovarian syndrome (PCOS) and functional hypothalamic amenorrhea. There are direct pharmacologic hormonal exposures, such as oral contraception and hormone replacement therapy, as well as potential hormonal changes related to diet composition, percent body fat, and body mass index. These hormonal variations potentially affect cardiovascular health through mechanisms that remain unclear. As one example, the Nurses' Health Study showed no cardiovascular risk reduction with ongoing hormone replacement therapy.[28] In contrast, it has been reported that elevated estradiol levels in men and women are associated with an increased risk of cardiac arrest, whereas higher testosterone levels are associated with a lower risk of cardiac arrest in men.[15]

It is not simply the addition or removal of hormones that influences cardiovascular risk in women. There is evidence that both deficiency and supplementation of hormones can influence CVD. The concomitant use of oral contraception and tobacco specifically increases the risk of developing hypertension as well as independently increasing the risk of CVD and venous thromboembolism.[29] PCOS, a state in which ovarian dysfunction results in the imbalance of reproductive hormones, is associated with metabolic syndrome (central obesity, insulin resistance, hypertension, and dyslipidemia with high triglycerides and/or low high-density lipoprotein), and a higher cardiovascular risk. Functional hypothalamic amenorrhea is associated with premature coronary atherosclerosis and a 50% increase in the risk of nonfatal and fatal heart disease. In this disease, the addition of oral contraceptives could be protective.

There are also direct hormonal effects notable on ECG tracings. Women have higher resting heart rates, shorter PR intervals, shorter atrial and AV node refractory periods, shorter QRS duration, a longer QT interval, and longer ventricular refractory periods. ECG changes can occur throughout the menstrual cycle. These physiological ECG changes can have an impact on the specificity of diagnostic cardiac testing, leads to greater sensitivity to QT-prolonging effect of medications, and increases the risk of torsades de pointes (especially during the follicular phase of the menstrual cycle) and other ventricular arrhythmias.

PREGNANCY-RELATED CONDITIONS: PREECLAMPSIA AND PERIPARTUM CARDIOMYOPATHY

Pregnancy itself places stress on the cardiovascular system. In addition, there are several conditions that increase lifetime risk of developing CVD.[11,30] Preeclampsia affects up to 8% of pregnancies and is thought to be the result of abnormal placentation. It is believed that during placentation, the spiral arteries fail to remodel, leading to hypoperfusion and hypoxemia. This triggers a systemic inflammatory response leading to endothelial dysfunction and vasoconstriction. The endpoint is maternal systemic hypertension and end-organ hypoperfusion directly affecting the fetus.[31] Preeclampsia is associated with pathophysiologic changes that increase short-term and long-term cardiovascular risks.[32] Diastolic left ventricular dysfunction occurs in preeclampsia in a manner that is similar to patients with essential hypertension. Preeclampsia is associated with a 6% to 12% cardiovascular complication rate that varies based on severity and the development of hemolysis, elevated liver enzymes, and thrombocytopenia syndrome.[33] The risk for major adverse cardiovascular events (including myocardial infarction) extends for at least 3 years postpartum.[33] Preeclampsia is a long-term risk factor for postpartum CVD.[32,33] Women with preeclamptic pregnancies are at a 2-fold increased risk of death from CVD.[34] In women who develop preeclampsia prior to 34 weeks of gestation, there is a 4-fold to 8-fold higher long-term mortality risk[35] that increases even further if a fetus is diagnosed with intrauterine growth restriction.[36] Identifying women with preeclampsia helps stratify long-term cardiovascular risk.

Other changes with potential cardiovascular impact in patients with preeclampsia include changes in lipoprotein profiles, the redistribution of visceral fat, and insulin resistance.[31] Because these changes are similar to those seen in patients with the metabolic syndrome, this might be the source of the increased cardiovascular risk associated with preeclampsia.[35] Changes in endothelial function noted in patients with preeclampsia are also seen in diabetes, smoking, and hypertension, which may promote premature atherosclerosis because of an increased tendency toward thrombosis, chronic inflammation, and plaque rupture.[35] Women with persistent hypertension after a diagnosis of preeclampsia are at higher long-term risk of developing CVD.[9]

Gestational diabetes mellitus (GDM) is also associated with a higher risk of subsequent CVD. Accelerated atherosclerosis, likely a manifestation of endothelial dysfunction, is associated with GDM.[13] Due to this risk, patients with a history of GDM should be screened for diabetes every 3 years.[9,37] Ultimately, up to 70% of women with GDM develop CVD within 30 years of pregnancy[9] even in the absence of overt diabetes mellitus.

PPCM occurs in patients with signs of systolic heart failure and no other identifiable cause from the last month of pregnancy through 4 weeks to 8 weeks postpartum. PPCM is associated with a mortality rate of 18% to 56%.[9] Therapy focuses on the safe and expedited delivery of the fetus and then incorporates usual management principles for systolic left ventricular dysfunction and congestive heart failure, bearing in mind any potential medication impact on lactation. Although 50% of patients recover normal left ventricular systolic function within 6 months, recurrence rates are high and associated morbidity is common. PPCM has a 20% to 30% risk of pulmonary edema and 14% risk of persistent left ventricular dysfunction.[38] In patients who recover normal left ventricular systolic function, there is a 20% chance of relapse with subsequent pregnancies. Patients in whom left ventricular ejection fraction does not improve have an overall mortality of 6% to 19%.[38,39] Contraception is important in patients with postpartum cardiomyopathy because of the risk of pregnancy to the mother and the potential teratogenicity of medications used for managing PPCM, including warfarin, angiotensin-converting enzyme inhibitors, or angiotensin receptor blockers. Estrogen-containing contraceptives are discouraged in PPCM patients because of an increased risk of QT prolongation and arrhythmias, particularly when used concurrently with heart failure medications.[38]

BREAST CANCER THERAPY AND CARDIOVASCULAR DISEASE

Because an aging population has higher rates of both CVD and breast cancer, recognizing and mitigating the late effects of breast cancer therapy are important to diminishing cardiovascular morbidity and improving long-term quality of life. Breast cancer therapies pose unique risks for CVD.[40] When choosing a treatment regimen, the underlying genetics and pathology of the breast cancer cell type and receptor status, staging, and recurrence rate of the primary tumor must be taken into account in the context of individual patient characteristics, such as age, existing CVD, and functional status to limit the cardiotoxic potential of chemotherapy. The possible effects of cancer therapy depend on the agent used and include new-onset hypertension, IHD (mediated by accelerated atherosclerosis and/or coronary artery vasospasm), cardiomyopathy, arterial thromboembolism (manifesting as angina, myocardial infarction, or stroke), and arrhythmias. Many patients with breast cancer also have independent risk factors for CVD.[41] Some risk factors for CVD, including obesity and tobacco use, concurrently increase the risk for breast cancer. Obesity, hypertension, and tobacco use potentiate the effects of chemotherapy on CVD.[41]

Among antineoplastic agents, the rates and mechanisms of cardiotoxicity differ widely. This is important when considering therapeutic options in the context of pre-existing cardiac risk factors to help determine which therapy is likely most effective with the lowest potential for side effects. Common agents, such as doxorubicin and trastuzumab, are associated with left ventricular systolic dysfunction, leading to heart failure. Other chemotherapeutic agents have a variety of cardiotoxic effects, including pericarditis, myocarditis, ventricular arrhythmias, bradycardia, endovascular damage, thrombosis, coronary vasospasm, ischemia, and hypertension.[42] There are 2 main types of chemotherapy-mediated cardiotoxicity: type I, in which irreversible myocyte necrosis occurs, and type II, in which potentially reversible myocyte stunning or hibernation may occur resulting in reversible cardiac contractile dysfunction.[40] Doxorubicin, an anthracycline with type I cardiotoxic potential, is associated with heart failure rates of 3% to 18% depending on the cumulative dose received. Incidence of cardiotoxicity increases with age, coexisting CVD and with prior mediastinal radiation.[42] Trastuzumab is associated with type II myocyte cardiotoxicity and a 2% to 4% risk of (typically reversible) heart failure.[42] Chemotherapy agents used sequentially or concurrently,[43] as in the use of tamoxifen with aromatase inhibitors, including anastrozole and letrozole, improve long-term survival with breast cancer but increase rates of hypercholesterolemia and thromboembolism.[42] Aromatase inhibitors increase the risk of arrhythmias, valvular heart disease, and pericarditis.[44] Early and consistent follow-up is important to allow cardiovascular risk factor modification, early diagnosis, and treatment while keeping in mind possible short-term and long-term consequences of chemotherapy.

Table 1 Pharmacotherapies for women		
Medication	Mortality Risk for Women	Side Effects in Women
Angiotensin-converting enzyme inhibitors	No mortality benefit in left ventricular dysfunction	More dry cough
Aspirin	Higher protection against stroke Lower protection against myocardial infarction	Greater bleeding risk
β-Blockers	More sensitive dose response for blood pressure and heart rate	No differences identified
Digoxin	Increased mortality	No differences identified
Statins	No differences	Higher incidence of myopathy

Radiation therapy is associated with a 0.2% to 3.5% increased risk of cardiovascular events in cancer survivors.[42] Preexisting hypertension and tobacco act synergistically to increase the incidence of fatal myocardial infarction in patients with a history of radiation therapy.[43] It is important to minimize the therapeutic field of radiation to limit cardiac exposure whenever possible to reduce subsequent risk. As with chemotherapeutic agents, cardiovascular toxicity in patients receiving radiation therapy depends on the exposed anatomy, cumulative dose and underlying patient characteristics.

Cardiac surveillance helps identify breast cancer patients likely to benefit from early diagnosis and treatment of left ventricular dysfunction, heart failure, atherosclerotic coronary disease, and valvular heart disease. Surveillance options include cardiac imaging with echocardiography or multiple gated acquisition scanning at regular intervals. Treatment of potential cardiotoxicity depends on the clinical presentation and patient functional status.[45–47]

GENDER DIFFERENCES IN PHARMACOTHERAPY

There are significant differences reported among certain pharmacotherapies for women compared with men, which may alter cardiovascular therapeutic choices for women (**Table 1**).

SUMMARY

CVD in women takes on many distinct forms. Understanding cardiac pathophysiology with an appreciation for distinct differences that occur in women improves the likelihood of accurate diagnosis. Nonocclusive coronary causes are more common compared with men. Specific cardiovascular pathophysiologies, including coronary microvascular dysfunction, coronary artery vasospasm, spontaneous coronary artery dissection, and stress-induced cardiomyopathy, are more common in women. Hormonal changes associated with the normal menstrual cycle, pregnancy, and menopause as well as other disease states affecting reproductive hormones, such as PCOS and hypothalamic amenorrhea, have a profound impact on when and how CVD presents in women. Obesity, tobacco use, and diabetes mellitus seem more potent cardiac risk factors in women. Additionally, breast cancer patients with ongoing or past treatment using radiation and/or potentially cardiotoxic chemotherapy are at risk for accelerated atherosclerosis and cardiac complications, the likelihood of which also depends on the presence of other traditional cardiac risk factors.

Women also have a higher prevalence of autoimmune and rheumatologic illnesses, which increases the risk of CVD. Women respond differently to physical and emotional stresses, which, coupled with specific personal, societal, and cultural factors, may uniquely increase an individual woman's risk for CVD. Pregnancy-related conditions, such as preeclampsia, gestational diabetes, and PPCM, are associated with higher rates of subsequent cardiovascular morbidity and mortality.

There is a need and opportunity for diagnostic and therapeutic modalities in CVD tailored distinctly to women. Early symptom recognition is the key to early diagnosis of CVD in women. When cardiovascular risk factors and symptoms are recognized early, women fare better when treated according to existing guidelines. Knowledge of the specific manifestations of CVD will ultimately lead to diminished health care disparities for women with CVD and improve global health.

REFERENCES

1. Merz CNB, Regitz-Zagrosek V. The case for sex- and gender-specific medicine. JAMA Intern Med 2014;174(8):1348–9.
2. Merz CNB. Sex, death, and the diagnosis gap. Circulation 2014;130:740–2.
3. Harvey RE, Coffman KE, Miller VM. Women-specific factors to consider in risk, diagnosis and treatment of cardiovascular disease. Womens Health 2015; 11(2):239–57.
4. Mehta LS, Beckie TM, DeVon HA, et al. Acute myocardial infarction in women: a scientific statement from the American Heart Association. Circulation 2016;133: 916–47.
5. McSweeney JC, Rosenfel AG, Abel WM, et al. Preventing and experiencing ischemic heart disease as a woman: state of the science, a scientific statement from the American Heart Association. Circulation 2016;133:1302–31.
6. Yihua L, Yun J, Dongshen Z. Coronary artery disease in premenopausal and postmenopausal women: risk factors, cardiovascular features, and recurrence. Int Heart J 2017;58(2):174–9.
7. Benjamin EJ, Blaha MJ, Chiuve SE, et al. Heart disease and stroke statistics-2017 update: a report from the American Heart Association. Circulation 2017;135: e1–459.
8. Merz CNB, Shaw LJ, Reis SE, et al. Insights from the NHLBI-sponsored women's ischemia syndrome evaluation (WISE) study: part II: gender differences in presentation, diagnosis, and outcome with regard to gender-based pathophysiology of atherosclerosis and macrovascular and microvascular coronary disease. J Cardiovasc Med 2006;47(3, suppl S):21S–9S.
9. Garcia M, Miller VM, Gulati M, et al. Focused cardiovascular care for women: the need and role in clinical practice. Mayo Clin Proc 2016;91(2):226–40.
10. Kothawade K, Merz CNB. Microvascular coronary dysfunction in women-pathophysiology, diagnosis, and management. Curr Probl Cardiol 2011;36: 291–318.
11. Pepine CJ. Ischemic heart disease in women. J Am Coll Cardiol 2006; 47(3,suppS):1S–3S.
12. Pepine CJ, Kerensky RA, Lambert CR, et al. Some thoughts on the vasculopathy of women with ischemic heart disease. J Am Coll Cardiol 2006;47(3):30S–4S.
13. Park K, Wei J, Minissian M, et al. Adverse pregnancy conditions, infertility and future cardiovascular risk: implications for mother and child. Cardiovasc Drugs Ther 2015;29(4):391–401.

14. Clegg D, Hevener AL, Moreau KL, et al. Sex hormones and cardiometabolic health: role of estrogen and estrogen receptors. Endocrinology 2017;158(5): 1095–105.

15. Gillis AM. Atrial fibrillation and ventricular arrhythmias: sex differences in electrophysiology, epidemiology, clinical presentation and clinical outcomes. Circulation 2017;135:593–608.

16. Crea F, Binder RK, Luscher TF. The year in cardiology 2016: acute coronary syndromes. Eur Heart J 2017;38:154–64.

17. Virani SS, Khan AN, Mendoza CE, et al. Takotsubo cardiomyopathy, or broken-heart syndrome. Tex Heart Inst J 2007;34:76–9.

18. Gottdiener JS, McClelland RL, Marshall R, et al. Outcome of congestive heart failure in elderly persons: influence of left ventricular systolic function: the cardiovascular health study. Ann Intern Med 2002;137(8):631–9.

19. Sedlak T, Izadnegahdar M, Humphries KH, et al. Sex-specific factors in microvascular angina. Can J Cardiol 2014;30:747–55.

20. Lew J, Sanghavi M, Ayers CR, et al. Sex-based differences in cardiometabolic biomarkers. Circulation 2017;135:544–55.

21. Gimenez MR, Reiter M, Twerenbold R, et al. Sex-specific chest pain characteristics in the early diagnosis of acute myocardial infarction. JAMA Intern Med 2014; 174(2):241–9.

22. Izadnegahdar M, Mackay M, Lee MK, et al. Sex and ethnic differences in outcomes of acute coronary syndrome and stable angina patients with obstructive coronary artery disease. Circ Cardiovasc Qual Outcomes 2016;9:S26–35.

23. Shaw LJ, Merz CNB, Pepine CJ, et al. Insights from the NHLBI-sponsored women's ischemia syndrome evaluation (WISE) study: part I: gender differences in traditional and novel risk factors, symptom evaluation, and gender-optimized diagnostic strategies. J Am Coll Cardiol 2006;47(3, suppl S):4S–20S.

24. Krantz DS, Olson MB, Francis JL, et al. Anger, hostility, and cardiac symptoms in women with suspected coronary artery disease: the women's ischemia syndrome evaluation (WISE) study. J Womens Health (Larchmt) 2006;15(10):1214–23.

25. Deo R, Vittinghoff E, Lin F, et al. Risk factor and prediction modeling for sudden cardiac death in women with coronary artery disease. Arch Intern Med 2011; 171(19):1703–9.

26. Gulati M, Shaw LJ, Merz CNB. Myocardial ischemia in women: lessons from the NHLBI WISE study. Clin Cardiol 2012;35(3):141–8.

27. Mann D, Zipes D, Libby P, et al. Barunwald's Heart Disease: A Textbook of Cardiovascular Medicine, Tenth Edition, Philadelphia: Elsevier; 2015.

28. Fazal L, Azibani F, Vodovar N, et al. Effects of biological sex on the pathophysiology of the heart. Br J Pharmacol 2017. https://doi.org/10.1111/bph.12279.

29. Sedlak T, Merz CNB, Shufelt C, et al. Contraception in patients with heart failure. Circulation 2012;126:1396–400.

30. Powe CE, Levine RJ, Karumanchi SA. Preeclampsia, a disease of the maternal endothelium: the role of antiangiogenic factors and implications for later cardiovascular disease. Circulation 2011;123:2856–69.

31. Wu P, Haththotuwa R, Kowk CS, et al. Preeclampsia and future cardiovascular health: a systematic review and meta-analysis. Circ Cardiovasc Qual Outcomes 2017;10:3003497.

32. Sanghavi M, Parikh NI. Harnessing the power of pregnancy and pregnancy-related events to predict cardiovascular disease in women. Circulation 2017; 135:590–2.

33. Melchiorre K, Sharma R, Thilaganathan B. Cardiovascular implications in pre-eclampsia: an overview. Circulation 2014;130:703–14.
34. Bokslag A, van Weissenbruch M, Mol BM, et al. Preeclampsia; short and long-term consequences for mother and neonate. Early Hum Dev 2016;35(4):470–3.
35. Cirillo PA, Cohn BA. Pregnancy complications and cardiovascular disease death: 50-year follow-up of the child health and development studies pregnancy cohort. Circulation 2015;132:1234–42.
36. Tanz LJ, Stuart JJ, Williams PL, et al. Preterm delivery and maternal cardiovascular disease in young women. Circulation 2017;135:578–89.
37. American College of Obstetrics and Gynecology. ACOG practice bulletin no. 137: gestational diabetes mellitus. Obstet Gynecol 2013;122(2 Pt1):406–16.
38. Lima FV, Yang J, Xu J, et al. National trends and in-hospital outcomes in pregnant women with heart disease in the United States. Am J Cardiol 2017;119(10): 1694–700.
39. Elkayam U, Tummala PP, Rao K, et al. Maternal and fetal outcomes of subsequent pregnancies in women with peripartum cardiomyopathy. N Engl J Med 2001;344: 1567–71.
40. Harbeck N, Ewer MS, De Laurentiis M, et al. Cardiovascular complications of conventional and targeted adjuvant breast cancer therapy. Ann Oncol 2011;22: 1250–8.
41. Maurea N, Coppola C, Ragone G, et al. Women survive breast cancer but fall victim to heart failure: the shadows and lights of targeted therapy. J Cardiovasc Med 2010;11:861–8.
42. Zagar TM, Cardinale DM, Marks LB. Breast cancer therapy-associated cardiovascular disease. Nat Rev Clin Oncol 2016;13:172–84.
43. Ky B, Vejpongsa P, Yeh ETH, et al. Emerging paradigms in cardiomyopathies associated with cancer therapies. Circ Res 2013;113:754–64.
44. Haque R, Shi J, Schottinger JE, et al. Cardiovascular disease after aromatase inhibitor use. JAMA Oncol 2016;2(12):1590–7.
45. Cadeddu C, Mercurio V, Spallarossa P, et al. Preventing antiblastic drug-related cardiomyopathy: old and new therapeutic strategies. J Cardiovasc Med 2016; 17(suppl1):e64–375.
46. Gulati G, Heck SL, Ree AH, et al. Prevention of cardiac dysfunction during adjuvant breast cancer therapy (PRADA): a 2 x 2 factorial, randomized, placebo-controlled, double-blind clinical trial of candesartan and metoprolol. Eur Heart J 2016;37:1671–80.
47. Tamargo J, Rosano G, Walther T, et al. Gender differences in the effects of cardiovascular drugs. Eur Heart J Cardiovasc Pharmacother 2017. https://doi.org/10.1093/3hjcvp/pvw042.

Heart Disease in Children

Richard U. Garcia, MD*, Stacie B. Peddy, MD

KEYWORDS

- Congenital heart disease • Children • Primary care • Cyanosis • Chest pain
- Heart murmur • Infective endocarditis

KEY POINTS

- Fetal and neonatal diagnosis of congenital heart disease (CHD) has improved the outcomes for children born with critical CHD.
- Treatment and management of CHD has improved significantly over the past 2 decades, allowing more children with CHD to grow into adulthood.
- Appropriate diagnosis and treatment of group A pharyngitis and Kawasaki disease in pediatric patients mitigate late complications.
- Chest pain, syncope, and irregular heart rhythm are common presentations in primary care. Although typically benign, red flag symptoms/signs should prompt a referral to cardiology for further evaluation.

INTRODUCTION

The modern incidence of congenital heart disease (CHD) has been reported at 6 to 11.1 per 1000 live births.[1,2] The true incidence is likely higher because many miscarriages are due to heart conditions incompatible with life. The unique physiology of CHD, the constantly developing nature of children, the differing presenting signs and symptoms, the multiple palliative or corrective surgeries, and the constant development of new strategies directed toward improving care in this population make pediatric cardiology an exciting field in modern medicine.

THE FETAL CIRCULATION AND TRANSITION TO NEONATAL LIFE

Cardiovascular morphogenesis is a complex process that transforms an initial single-tube heart to a 4-chamber heart with 2 separate outflow tracts. Multiple and

Disclosure Statement: All Authors take responsibility for all aspects of the reliability and freedom from bias of the information presented and their discussed interpretation. No conflict of interest, grants, or other financial support was received for this article.
Division of Cardiac Critical Care Medicine, Departments of Pediatrics and Critical Care Medicine, The University of Pennsylvania and the Children's Hospital of Philadelphia, 34th Street, Civic Center Boulevard, Philadelphia, PA 19104, USA
* Corresponding author.
E-mail address: rugsal25@gmail.com

overlapping signaling events make this possible and when the process deviates from normal, CHD occurs.[3] The fetal circulation occurs in a parallel circuit. Because the source of oxygenation in fetal life is the placenta, only 10% of the combined cardiac output reaches the fetal lungs.[4] Because of a mechanism of preferential blood flow streaming, the oxygenated blood coming back from the placenta bypasses the liver through the ductus venosum, enters the right atrium by the inferior vena cavae, and is streamed through the patent foramen ovale to the left atria, providing the brain with highly oxygenated blood. Only approximately 10% of the combined cardiac output goes through the aortic isthmus to the descending aorta. Fetal systemic venous return enters the right atrium through the superior and inferior vena cavae and streams toward the tricuspid valve to reach the pulmonary artery, subsequently crossing the patent ductus arteriosus almost in its entirety (approximately 50% of the combined cardiac output) to reach the placenta through the descending aorta.[4]

These unique characteristics of the fetal circulation allow for tolerance of complex heart disease like hypoplastic left heart syndrome in utero with minimal hemodynamic consequences. The extra utero circulation, however, occurs in parallel. Once a fetus takes that important first breath, a cascade of events leads to significant hemodynamic changes, making tolerance of complex CHD difficult.

SCREENING FOR CONGENITAL HEART DISEASE: WHEN AND WHO?

The etiology of CHD is multifactorial. Prenatal diagnosis of critical neonatal CHD affects neonatal morbidity and (to a lesser extent), mortality.[5] Accurate prenatal diagnosis also contributes to preservation of long-term neurocognitive function and outcome,[6] highlighting the importance of accurate prenatal screening and prompt diagnosis. The risk for CHD in the general population is less than 1% and in this setting, fetal echocardiography screening is not recommended. If, however, the risk for CHD is greater than 3% (**Table 1**), fetal echocardiography should be performed. When the risk for CHD is estimated at 1% to 2%, fetal echocardiography can be considered, although the relative benefit of such additional testing in this population is not clear. In all cases, fetuses with an abnormal screening ultrasound of the heart should have a detailed fetal echocardiogram read by a trained examiner.[5]

Kemper and colleagues[7] made recommendations for universal neonatal screening to diagnose critical CHD (CCHD). These recommendations included measurement of the percutaneous oxygen saturation in the right hand and feet between 24 hours to 48 hours of birth or just before discharge if a neonate leaves the hospital before 24 hours of life.

A screen is positive screening if

- The oxygen saturation is below 90% in the right hand OR feet during 3 consecutive measurements separated by 1 hour.
- The oxygen saturation is below 95% and above 90% in the right hand AND feet OR more than a 3% difference between the right hand and feet saturation during 3 consecutive measurements separated by 1 hour.

The screen is negative if

- The oxygen saturation is above 95% in the right hand OR feet AND less than a 3% difference between the right hand and feet saturation at any point during 3 consecutive measurements separated by 1 hour.

These recommendations were endorsed by American Academy of Pediatrics, the American College of Cardiology Foundation, and the American Heart Association

Table 1
Common risk factors for congenital heart disease

Risk Factors	Absolute Risk, Percent of Live Births	Level of Evidence	Timing/Frequency of Evaluation
Pregestational diabetes	3–5	I/A	18–22 wk. Repeat evaluation in third trimester if hemoglobulin A_{1c} >6% may be considered
Gestational diabetes, hemoglobulin A_{1c} <6%	<1	III/B	If hemoglobulin A_{1c} >6%, evaluation in third trimester to evaluate for ventricular hypertrophy
Phenylketonuria 10–12 (preconception metabolic control may affect risk)	12–14	I/A	18–22 wk. Only if periconception phenylalanine level >10 mg/dL
Vitamin K antagonists	<1	III/B	Not indicated
Lupus or Sjögren syndrome only if SSA/SSB autoantibody positive	1–5	IIa/B	16 wk, then weekly or every other wk to 28 wk
Lithium	<2	IIb/B	18–22 wk first-trimester exposure
Use of assisted reproduction technology	1.1–3.3	IIa/A	18–22 wk
Maternal structural cardiac disease	3–7	I/B	18–22 wk
Paternal structural cardiac disease	2–3	I/B	18–22 wk
Sibling with structural cardiac disease	3 8 for hypoplastic left heart syndrome	I/B	18–22 wk

Data from Donofrio MT, Moon-Grady AJ, Hornberger LK, et al. Diagnosis and treatment of fetal cardiac disease: a scientific statement from the American Heart Association. Circulation 2014;129(21):2183–242.

(AHA) Council on Cardiovascular Disease in the Young and the screening algorithm added to the US Recommended Uniform Screening Panel in 2011. Any newborn with a positive screen and no clear clinical picture to explain the hypoxemia should be suspected of having CCHD and should undergo a diagnostic echocardiogram read by a pediatric cardiologist. Consultation with a pediatric cardiologist is recommended, when feasible, before obtaining the echocardiogram.[7]

Currently, screening for CCHD has been adopted in most developed countries. In the United States, 46 states and the District of Columbia include screening for CCHD as part of their routine newborn screening programs. Using this CCHD screening protocol, it is estimated that 875 infants with CCHDs are detected annually in the United States.[8] The recommended protocol has a low sensitivity to detect coarctation of the aorta, a common cause of CCHD,[9,10] necessitating the need to maintain vigilance for clinical signs and/or symptoms of CCHD, especially during the first weeks of life.

DUCTAL-DEPENDENT CRITICAL CONGENITAL HEART DISEASE

The ductus arteriosus functionally closes during the first 24 hours to 72 hours after birth. This is potentially after discharge from the newborn nursery. Patients with CCHD can, therefore, present to their primary care provider undiagnosed and with impending signs or symptoms of severe cyanosis or critical systemic hypoperfusion. These early signs and symptoms of CCHD are variable and nonspecific, including tachypnea, irritability, cyanosis, severe pallor, increased precordial activity, poor peripheral pulses, prolong capillary refill, and feeding intolerance. If CCHD is suspected based on any of these parameters, prompt transport to an appropriate facility for fluid resuscitation, rapid initiation of intravenous prostaglandins, and early consultation with pediatric cardiology are important.

ROUTINE WELL-CHILD CHECKUP: WHO NEEDS TO SEE A PEDIATRIC CARDIOLOGIST?

Well-child visits provide an opportunity to follow patients closely over time. In the context of the patient-centered medical home, they provide an opportunity to detect signs or symptoms of heart disease affecting normal development.

History

During every routine visit, a detailed past medical history (including cardiovascular history) and past family history should be obtained. Important cardiovascular symptoms include chest pain, syncope, palpitations, exercise tolerance, and feeding tolerance. Infants with pulmonary overcirculation take longer to complete each feed, work harder to feed, and often exhibit signs and symptoms during feeding. Therefore, especially in infancy, a detailed feeding history is important. This history should include the volume of each feed, the number of feeds per day, the amount of time required to complete each feed, and the presence of diaphoresis, cyanosis, or difficulty with latching or suckling.

Vital Signs (Including the Growth Chart)

Vital signs are a cornerstone element of each routine visit. Values should be compared with normative standards, which vary by age. Oxygen saturation can help exclude subclinical hypoxemia, 4-extremity blood pressure (BP) measurement can help diagnose coarctation of the aorta, unexplained tachycardia or tachypnea can be early presenting signs of myocarditis or cardiomyopathy, and persistent unexplained low-grade fevers can raise concern for endocarditis in patients with known risk factors. It is equally important to accurately measure and record growth during well-child visits. A drop of 2 weight percentiles between visits is considered abnormal and should be investigated. Although the differential diagnosis of failure to thrive is extensive, CHD should be considered a potential cause.

Physical Examination—Murmurs are Common

Many physical findings are particular to the pediatric cardiovascular examination. On inspection, jugular venous distention is rare, even in children with overt heart failure. Chest skeletal deformities like pectus excavatum or carinatum may be noticed and warrant further investigation. On palpation, the presence of musculoskeletal chest pain is common in healthy individuals. Abdominal tenderness and/or pain is a common presenting symptom in children with heart failure. On auscultation, murmurs are common in children (**Table 2**). At least 50% of children have a heart murmur during their lifetime.[11] Despite the general association of murmurs to CHD, most of the murmurs in the pediatric population are innocent, with no

Table 2
Common innocent murmurs

	Clinical Characteristics	Usual Age of Presentation	Common Natural Course
Peripheral pulmonary stenosis	Grade 1–2, low-pitched, midsystolic ejection murmur. Louder over the second left intercostal space with radiation to the axilla and back.	Neonate	Disappears by 3–6 mo of age
Stills murmur	Grade 1–3, low-frequency systolic murmur. Louder left lower sternal border. Has classic vibratory or musical quality. Louder supine and softer when patient is in the sitting position.	Toddlers to adolescent age	Disappears by adolescent age
Cervical venous hum	Grade 1–3 low-pitched continuous murmur but louder in diastole. Louder over anterior neck lateral to the sternocleidomastoid muscle. Softer or disappearance when turning neck or supine position.	Toddlers to 8–10 y	Disappears by early adolescent years

clinical implication. Usually, innocent heart murmurs change or disappear with position changes (supine to sitting or vice versa), are systolic, tend to disappear and reappear (for example during febrile emergency room visit or anemia), and are associated with normal vital signs, growth, and development.[12] Unlike adults, a third heart sound is common in healthy children (although it may be associated with congestive heart failure in selected patients). The presence of a click is indicative of structural heart disease and usually has a higher pitch compared with other heart sounds.[12]

COMMON CHIEF COMPLAINTS IN THE OFFICE: CHEST PAIN, SYNCOPE, AND IRREGULAR HEART RHYTHM

Chest pain is one of the most common reasons for consultation with a pediatric cardiologist. This is often driven by parental anxiety because chest pain is associated with significant morbidity and mortality in the adult population. A review of a decade of pediatric cardiology chest pain referrals at Boston Children's Hospital (approximately 18,000 patient years) revealed that only 1% (n = 3700) of the patients had a cardiac etiology for their chest pain and that no patient discharged from the clinic with a diagnosis of noncardiac chest pain died because of a cardiac condition over an average follow-up period of 4.4 years (range: 0.5–10.4 years).[13]

In the primary care setting, red flags that warrant further referral to pediatric cardiology are family history of sudden death, history of CHD or heart transplant, history of syncope with exercise, history of palpitations, chest pain during exercise, and an abnormal ECG. Symptoms and signs that reassuring of a noncardiac etiology included robust exercise tolerance, nonexertional chest pain, reproduction of chest pain with palpation, pain that worsens with inspiration, pain related to food intake, and pain that changes locations within or across the chest.

Syncope is another frequent reason for consultation in the pediatric age group. With syncope, parents are typically concern about sudden cardiac death. Syncope is common in pediatrics, with peak incidence in 9 year olds and 14 year olds, and peaks again in 15 year olds to 19 year olds, with the second peak more common in female patients.[14,15] The most common cause of pediatric syncope is neurocardiogenic (vasovagal syncope [VVS]) accounting for 75% to 80% of cases.[15] VVS typically includes prodromal symptoms like nausea, vomiting, dizziness, lightheadedness, and blurry vision before the syncopal event followed by quick recovery to baseline. Additionally, VVS patients often have a history of poor hydration and exertion in hot weather. Red flags for syncope included syncope with no prodromal symptoms, sudden collapse (usually during exertion), family history of sudden unexplained death, and abnormal ECG (in particular QT interval abnormalities), a systolic murmur that intensifies with the Valsalva maneuver on physical examination, gallop rhythm, and unexplained tachycardia. Patients presenting to the office with red flags should be restricted from exercise pending a prompt cardiology evaluation.

Irregular heart rhythms are occasionally noted during routine pediatric examinations. This is a common physiologic phenomenon known as sinus arrhythmia — the reflexive heart rate change with the respiratory cycle due to children having a strong vagal tone and high baroreceptor reflex sensitivity.[16] During inspiration, the vagal tone decreases with subsequent increase in the heart rate while expiration restores vagal tone and decreases heart rate. The differential diagnosis of sinus arrhythmia includes premature atrial contractions and atrioventricular node block. In general, this finding is innocuous and can be managed with simple reassurance.

SYSTEMIC HYPERTENSION: SCREENING AND MANAGEMENT

Hypertension is underdiagnosed in children. The importance of early diagnosis and management is to prevent end-organ damage (eg, left ventricular hypertrophy, retinopathy, and renal damage), address treatable causes of secondary hypertension, and, to some extent, reduce adulthood hypertension because several studies have shown linear correlation between childhood and adult hypertension.[17] The "Fourth Report on the Diagnosis, Evaluation, and Treatment of High Blood Pressure in Children and Adolescents" published by the National Heart, Lung, and Blood Institute[18] recommends accurately measuring and recording BP for all children older than 3 years of age during routine clinic visits (**Table 3**). Pediatric BP should be measured via auscultation of the right arm using an appropriate-sized cuff.[18]

Normative percentiles of BP averaged over 3 different measurement occasions provide accurate categorization, according to either the systolic or diastolic BP percentile (whichever is higher).[18]

DYSLIPIDEMIA SCREENING AND MANAGEMENT

Dyslipidemia is a multifactorial condition involving elevation of total cholesterol, low-density lipoprotein (LDL) and triglycerides, with lower levels of high-density lipoprotein. The link between dyslipidemia and cardiovascular disease is well established in adults. In children, however, the association of dyslipidemia and cardiovascular disease is not as clear. Whether early detection and management of dyslipidemia decreases the incidence of ischemic disease in young adults is under debate. Currently, the American Academy of Pediatrics recommends universal lipid screening between ages 9 years and 11 years and again between ages 17 years and 21 years. These guidelines also recommend selective screening for children older than 2 years old based on based on individual risk factors.[19] The US Preventive Services Task Force (USPSTF), however, suggests that the current evidence in the literature is insufficient to assess the balance of benefits and harms

Table 3
Fourth report recommendations for diagnosis and management of pediatric systemic hypertension[a]

	Systolic Blood Pressure or Diastolic Blood Pressure Percentile for Age, Gender, and Height	Treatment	Further Management
Normal	<90th percentile	Weight management, encourage physical activity and healthy diet.	Follow-up during next routine visit
Prehypertension	90th–<95th percentile	Weight management, encourage physical activity and healthy diet.	Remeasure in 6 mo
Stage I hypertension	95th–99th percentile + 5 mm Hg	Weight management, encourage physical activity and healthy diet. Initiate pharmacologic therapy if risk factors present.[a]	Recheck in 1–2 wk or sooner if a patient is symptomatic; if persistently elevated on 2 additional occasions, evaluate[b] or refer to source of care within 1 mo.
Stage II hypertension	>99th percentile + 5 mm Hg	Weight management, encourage physical activity and healthy diet. Initiate pharmacologic therapy.	Evaluate[b] or refer to source of care within 1 wk or immediately if the patient is symptomatic.

[a] Risk factors: symptomatic hypertension, secondary hypertension, target organ damage, diabetes mellitus (types 1 and 2), and persistent hypertension despite nonpharmacologic measures.
[b] Initial evaluation includes detailed family and past medical history, blood urea nitrogen, creatinine, electrolytes, urinalysis, urine culture, complete blood cell count, renal ultrasound, fasting lipid panel and glucose, echocardiogram, retinal examination, and drug screen test.

of screening for lipid disorders in children and adolescents 20 years or younger and has recommended against universal screening.[20]

A primary step in treating childhood dyslipidemia is instituting the Cardiovascular Health Integrated Lifestyle Diet. This can be facilitated with the help of a nutritionist. Pharmacologic therapy is recommended for children with no risk factors if their LDL is over 190 mg/dL and for children with LDL greater than 130 mg/dL if they have multiple risk factors and/or their triglycerides level is over 500 mg/dL.[19]

ENDOCARDITIS IN CHILDREN

In 2007, the AHA modified their infective endocarditis prophylaxis guidelines (**Box 1**). Indications for prophylaxis were reduced for dental procedures (**Table 4**) and genitourinary and gastrointestinal tract procedures.[21]

An expanding number of surgical procedures and improvements in materials have contributed to an increasing number of children with CHD surviving the neonatal period. With this, there have been no significant changes in the trend of infective endocarditis diagnosis or hospitalization in children with the revised prophylaxis guidelines over 11 years.[22]

Box 1
Cardiac conditions associated with the highest risk of adverse outcome from endocarditis for which prophylaxis with dental procedures is reasonable

Prosthetic cardiac valve or prosthetic material used for cardiac valve repair

Previous infective endocarditis

CHD[a]
    Unrepaired cyanotic CHD, including palliative shunts and conduits
    Completely repaired congenital heart defect with prosthetic material or device, whether placed by surgery or by catheter intervention, during the first 6 months after the procedure[b]
    Repaired CHD with residual defects at the site or adjacent to the site of a prosthetic patch or prosthetic device (which inhibit endothelialization)

Cardiac transplantation recipients who develop cardiac valvulopathy

[a] Except for the conditions listed, antibiotic prophylaxis is no longer recommended for any other form of CHD.

[b] Prophylaxis is reasonable because endothelialization of prosthetic material occurs within 6 months after the procedure.

From Wilson W, Taubert KA, Gewitz M, et al. Prevention of infective endocarditis: guidelines from the American Heart Association: a guideline from the American Heart Association Rheumatic Fever, Endocarditis, and Kawasaki Disease Committee, Council on Cardiovascular Disease in the Young, and the Council on Clinical Cardiology, Council on Cardiovascular Surgery and Anesthesia, and the Quality of Care and Outcomes Research Interdisciplinary Working Group. Circulation 2007;116(15):1745; with permission.

Table 4
Regimens for dental procedure

Situation	Agent	Regimen: Single Dose 30–60 Minutes before Procedure	
		Adults	Children
Oral	Amoxicillin	2 g	50 mg/kg
Unable to take oral medication	Ampicillin OR Cefazolin or ceftriaxone	2 g IM or IV 1 g IM or IV	50 mg/kg IM or IV 50 mg/kg IM or IV
Allergic to penicillins or ampicillin—oral	Cephalexin[a,b] OR Clindamycin OR Azithromycin or clarithromycin	2 g 600 mg 500 mg	50 mg/kg 20 mg/kg 15 mg/kg
Allergic to penicillins or ampicillin and unable to take oral medication	Cefazolin or ceftriaxone[b] OR Clindamycin	1 g IM or IV 600 mg IM or IV	50 mg/kg IM or IV 20 mg/kg IM or IV

Abbreviations: IM, intramuscular; IV, intravenous.
[a] Or other first-generation or second-generation oral cephalosporin in equivalent adult or pediatric dosage.
[b] Cephalospoins should not be used in an individual with a history of anaphylaxis, angioedema, or urticaria with penicillins or ampicillin.
From Wilson W, Taubert KA, Gewitz M, et al. Prevention of infective endocarditis: guidelines from the American Heart Association: a guideline from the American Heart Association Rheumatic Fever, Endocarditis, and Kawasaki Disease Committee, Council on Cardiovascular Disease in the Young, and the Council on Clinical Cardiology, Council on Cardiovascular Surgery and Anesthesia, and the Quality of Care and Outcomes Research Interdisciplinary Working Group. Circulation 2007;116(15):1747; with permission.

KAWASAKI DISEASE

The etiology of Kawasaki disease (KD), a self-limiting systemic vasculitis first described in 1967 by Dr Tomisaku Kawasaki, remains elusive.[23] KD most commonly affects children between ages 6 months and 5 years and rarely occurs beyond childhood.[24] The diagnosis of classic KD is based on clinical criteria and includes fever for at least 5 days and at least 4 of the following:

- Bilateral conjunctivae injection (usually with no eye discharge)
- Mucous membranes changes: injected pharynx, fissured lips, and strawberry tongue
- Polymorphous rash
- Peripheral extremity changes: edema, erythema, and periungual desquamation
- Cervical adenopathy; usually unilateral

Coronary artery aneurysm are of particular concern in patients with KD. Studies using high-resolution echocardiography indicate that at least 10% of children who ultimately develop coronary artery aneurysms do not meet the criteria for classic KD.[25] For this reason, incomplete KD has been introduced as a diagnosis. In children having at least 5 days of fever and at least 2 additional classic clinical findings, further evaluation by high-definition echocardiography and laboratory testing is indicated.[26] Treatment with intravenous immunoglobulin and high-dose aspirin have converted the disease from one associated with persistent coronary artery aneurysms in 20% to 25% of patients and mortality in up to 2% to a one that is fully curable in as many as 98% of children.[27] If KD is suspected based on clinical findings, prompt referral leads to timely diagnosis, appropriate management, and improved outcomes.

GROUP A STREPTOCOCCUS PHARYNGITIS: PREVENTING ACUTE RHEUMATIC FEVER AND RHEUMATIC HEART DISEASE

The incidence of acute rheumatic fever (ARF) and rheumatic heart disease (RHD) has declined in most developed nations. Group A streptococcus (GAS) pharyngitis remains common, however, in routine clinical practice. Most children affected by GAS pharyngitis are 5 years to 15 years of age. Clinical findings suggestive of GAS pharyngitis include sore throat (generally of sudden onset), pain on swallowing, fever of varying degree, headache, abdominal pain, nausea, and vomiting. Additional clinical findings include tonsillopharyngeal erythema with or without exudates, anterior cervical lymphadenitis, soft palate petechiae, beefy red swollen uvula, and a scarlatiniform rash.[28] The appropriate identification and treatment of GAS pharyngitis reduces the incidence of ARF/RHD as known sequelae.[28,29] For multiple reasons, including access to health care, not all cases of ARF/RHD can be prevented. In 2015, the AHA modified the Jones criteria for the diagnosis of ARF to better reflect the changing epidemiology of the disease (**Table 5**). Specifically, the AHA established distinct diagnostic criteria for low-risk populations ($\leq$2/100,000 school-aged children) and moderate-risk to high-risk (>2/100,000 school-aged children) populations.[30] A diagnosis of initial ARF requires 2 major criteria or 1 major plus 2 minor criteria. A diagnosis of recurrent ARF requires either 2 major criteria, 1 major and 2 minor criteria, or 3 minor criteria.[30]

Some cases of ARF present with severe manifestations, including acute mitral and/or aortic insufficiency and heart failure. Therefore, in patients with suspected ARF, expeditious referral to a tertiary care center is appropriate. Additionally, patients who have had 1 episode of ARF require long-term pediatric cardiology follow-up to

Table 5
The American Heart Association 2015 modified Jones criteria for the diagnosis of acute rheumatic fever

Increased or rising anti-streptolysin O titer or other streptococcal antibodies (anti-DNASE B) (class I; level of evidence B) or
A positive throat culture for group A β-hemolytic streptococci (class I; level of evidence B) or
A positive rapid GAD carbohydrate antigen test in a child whose clinical presentation suggests a high pretest probability of streptococcal pharyngitis (class I; level of evidence B).

	Major Criteria	Minor Criteria
Low-risk population	Carditis (clinical and/or echocardiographic) Arthritis (polyarthritis only) Chorea Erythema marginatum Subcutaneous nodules	Polyarthralgia Fever ($\geq$38.5°C) Erythrocyte sedimentation rate $\geq$60 mm/h and/or C-reactive protein $\geq$3.0 mg/dL Prolonged PR interval, after accounting for age variability (unless carditis is a major criterion)
Moderate-risk and high-risk populations	Carditis (clinical and/or echocardiographic) Arthritis (including monoarthritis, polyarthritis, or polyarthralgia) Chorea Erythema marginatum Subcutaneous nodules	Monoarthralgia Fever ($\geq$38.5°C) Erythrocyte sedimentation rate $\geq$30 mm/h and/or C-reactive protein $\geq$3.0 mg/dL Prolonged PR interval, after accounting for age variability (unless carditis is a major criterion)

Data from Gewitz MH, Baltimore RS, Tani LY, et al. Revision of the Jones Criteria for the diagnosis of acute rheumatic fever in the era of Doppler echocardiography: a scientific statement from the American Heart Association. Circulation 2015;131(20):1806-18.

prevent recurrence (typically long-term antibiotic prophylaxis) even without cardiac involvement during the initial episode.

THE ROLE OF PRIMARY CARE IN CHILDREN WITH HEART TRANSPLANTATIONS

The first human heart transplantation was successfully performed by Christiaan Barnard in 1967. Infant heart transplantation was first attempted the same year. The first successful neonatal heart transplant took place in 1985. The number of infant and pediatric heart transplantations has since gradually increased.[31] Caring for children before and after heart transplantation requires a multidisciplinary team, including a central role for primary care. The pretransplant period should be used to ensure that patients are up to date on immunizations. Live vaccines can be given up to 4 weeks before transplant, and for patients on the heart transplant list, the mumps-measles-rubella and varicella vaccines can be given as early as 6 months of age.[32] In post-transplant patients, only nonlive vaccines are recommended. For patients traveling in areas endemic for typhoid fever, the inactivated polysaccharide typhoid vaccine is recommended if a patient is traveling for long periods of time or planning to engage in extended outdoor activities. The live oral typhoid vaccine and the live attenuated yellow fever vaccine are contraindicated. The BCG vaccine is a live attenuated *Mycobacterium bovis*–derived vaccine and is also contraindicated in immunocompromised individuals.[33]

Early signs of a possible rejection are important to identify in the primary care setting as well. These include increased baseline heart rate, abdominal pain, rash, diarrhea, nausea, vomiting, and decreased exercise tolerance (especially if suspicion for infection is low). On physical examination, signs of rejection include unexplained tachycardia, new murmur, gallop rhythm (+S3), hepatomegaly, pulmonary crackles, and poor peripheral perfusion. If rejection is suspected, the heart transplant team should be contacted immediately.

REFERENCES

1. Hoffman JI, Kaplan S. The incidence of congenital heart disease. J Am Coll Cardiol 2002;39(12):1890–900.
2. Qu Y, Liu X, Zhuang J, et al. Incidence of congenital heart disease: the 9-year experience of the guangdong registry of congenital heart disease, China. PLoS One 2016;11(7):e0159257.
3. Gittenberger-de Groot AC, Bartelings MM, Poelmann RE, et al. Embryology of the heart and its impact on understanding fetal and neonatal heart disease. Semin Fetal Neonatal Med 2013;18(5):237–44.
4. Rudolph AM. Congenital diseases of the heart: clinical-physiological considerations. Chichester, United Kingdom: Wiley-Blackwell; 2009.
5. Donofrio MT, Moon-Grady AJ, Hornberger LK, et al. Diagnosis and treatment of fetal cardiac disease: a scientific statement from the American Heart Association. Circulation 2014;129(21):2183–242.
6. Kipps AK, Feuille C, Azakie A, et al. Prenatal diagnosis of hypoplastic left heart syndrome in current era. Am J Cardiol 2011;108(3):421–7.
7. Kemper AR, Mahle WT, Martin GR, et al. Strategies for implementing screening for critical congenital heart disease. Pediatrics 2011;128(5):e1259–67.
8. Ailes EC, Gilboa SM, Honein MA, et al. Estimated number of infants detected and missed by critical congenital heart defect screening. Pediatrics 2015;135(6):1000–8.
9. Oster ME, Kochilas L. Screening for critical congenital heart disease. Clin Perinatol 2016;43(1):73–80.
10. Oster ME, Aucott SW, Glidewell J, et al. Lessons learned from newborn screening for critical congenital heart defects. Pediatrics 2016;137(5):e20154573.
11. Allen HD, Shaddy RE, Penny DJ, et al. Moss and Adams' heart disease in infants, children, and adolescents: including the fetus and young adult. Philadelphia: Wolters Kluwer; 2016.
12. Mesropyan L, Sanil Y. Innocent heart murmurs from the perspective of the pediatrician. Pediatr Ann 2016;45(8):e306–9.
13. Saleeb SF, Li WY, Warren SZ, et al. Effectiveness of screening for life-threatening chest pain in children. Pediatrics 2011;128(5):e1062–8.
14. McLeod KA. Syncope in childhood. Arch Dis Child 2003;88(4):350–3.
15. Friedman KG, Alexander ME. Chest pain and syncope in children: a practical approach to the diagnosis of cardiac disease. J Pediatr 2013;163(3):896–901.e891-3.
16. Wagner GS, Strauss DG. Marriott's practical electrocardiography. Philadelphia: Wolters Kluwer Health/Lippincott Williams & Wilkins; 2014.
17. Rao G. Diagnosis, epidemiology, and management of hypertension in children. Pediatrics 2016;138(2).
18. National High Blood Pressure Education Program Working Group on High Blood Pressure in Children Adolescents. The fourth report on the diagnosis, evaluation, and treatment of high blood pressure in children and adolescents. Pediatrics 2004;114(2 Suppl 4th Report):555–76.

19. Expert Panel on Integrated Guidelines for Cardiovascular Health and Risk Reduction in Children and Adolescents National Heart, Lung, and Blood Institute. Expert panel on integrated guidelines for cardiovascular health and risk reduction in children and adolescents: summary report. Pediatrics 2011;128(Suppl 5):S213–56.

20. US Preventive Services Task Force, Bibbins-Domingo K, Grossman DC, et al. Screening for lipid disorders in children and adolescents: US preventive services task force recommendation statement. JAMA 2016;316(6):625–33.

21. Wilson W, Taubert KA, Gewitz M, et al. Prevention of infective endocarditis: guidelines from the American Heart Association: a guideline from the American Heart Association rheumatic fever, endocarditis, and kawasaki disease committee, council on cardiovascular disease in the young, and the council on clinical cardiology, council on cardiovascular surgery and anesthesia, and the quality of care and outcomes research interdisciplinary working group. Circulation 2007; 116(15):1736–54.

22. Bates KE, Hall M, Shah SS, et al. Trends in infective endocarditis hospitalisations at United States children's hospitals from 2003 to 2014: impact of the 2007 American Heart Association antibiotic prophylaxis guidelines. Cardiol Young 2017; 27(4):686–90.

23. Kawasaki T. Acute febrile mucocutaneous syndrome with lymphoid involvement with specific desquamation of the fingers and toes in children. Arerugi 1967; 16(3):178–222 [in Japanese].

24. Nakamura Y, Yashiro M, Uehara R, et al. Epidemiologic features of Kawasaki disease in Japan: results of the 2009-2010 nationwide survey. J Epidemiol 2012;22(3):216–21.

25. Sundel RP. Update on the treatment of Kawasaki disease in childhood. Curr Rheumatol Rep 2002;4(6):474–82.

26. Newburger JW, Takahashi M, Gerber MA, et al. Diagnosis, treatment, and long-term management of Kawasaki disease: a statement for health professionals from the committee on rheumatic fever, endocarditis and kawasaki disease, council on cardiovascular disease in the young, American Heart Association. Circulation 2004;110(17):2747–71.

27. Cohen E, Sundel R. Kawasaki disease at 50 years. JAMA Pediatr 2016;170(11): 1093–9.

28. Gerber MA, Baltimore RS, Eaton CB, et al. Prevention of rheumatic fever and diagnosis and treatment of acute Streptococcal pharyngitis: a scientific statement from the American Heart Association rheumatic fever, endocarditis, and kawasaki disease committee of the council on cardiovascular disease in the young, the interdisciplinary council on functional genomics and translational biology, and the interdisciplinary council on quality of care and outcomes research: endorsed by the American Academy of Pediatrics. Circulation 2009;119(11):1541–51.

29. Carapetis JR, Beaton A, Cunningham MW, et al. Acute rheumatic fever and rheumatic heart disease. Nat Rev Dis Primers 2016;2:15084.

30. Gewitz MH, Baltimore RS, Tani LY, et al. Revision of the Jones criteria for the diagnosis of acute rheumatic fever in the era of Doppler echocardiography: a scientific statement from the American Heart Association. Circulation 2015;131(20):1806–18.

31. Bailey LL. Origins of neonatal heart transplantation: an historical perspective. Semin Thorac Cardiovasc Surg Pediatr Card Surg Annu 2011;14(1):98–100.

32. Abuali MM, Arnon R, Posada R. An update on immunizations before and after transplantation in the pediatric solid organ transplant recipient. Pediatr Transpl 2011;15(8):770–7.

33. Lopez MJ, Thomas S. Immunization of children after solid organ transplantation. Pediatr Clin North Am 2003;50(6):1435–49, ix-x.

Cardiac Imaging Modalities and Appropriate Use

Paul Gabriel Peterson, MD[a,b,*], Michael Berge, MD[c],
John P. Lichtenberger III, MD[b], Maureen N. Hood, PhD[a],
Vincent B. Ho, MD, MBA[a,b]

KEYWORDS

- Cardiac imaging • CMR • CCTA • CAC • Appropriate use

KEY POINTS

- Advanced cardiac imaging modalities to include calcium scoring computed tomography (CT), coronary CT angiography (CCTA), and cardiac MRI (CMR) are increasing in availability and accessibility.
- Awareness of the fundamentals for each of these imaging techniques, unique imaging challenges, and appropriate use criteria is critical for ordering physicians and providers.
- CCTA is a rapid examination with numerous radiation dose optimization and contrast dose reduction strategies available with appropriate patient preparation.
- CMR is a flexible cardiac imaging modality with no ionizing radiation patient exposure concerns, which can be tailored to answer multiple clinical questions, including structure, morphology, function, viability, and flow analysis.

Video content accompanies this article at http://www.primarycare.theclinics. com.

Disclaimer: The views expressed in this article are those of the authors and do not reflect the official policy of the Department of Army, Navy, Air Force or the US Government.
Disclosure Statement: P.G. Peterson, M. Berge, and J.P. Lichtenberger have no disclosures. M.N. Hood and V.B. Ho receive in-kind research support from GE Healthcare.
[a] Department of Radiology, Walter Reed National Military Medical Center, 8901 Rockville Pike, Building 9, 1st Floor, Bethesda, MD 20889, USA; [b] Department of Radiology and Radiological Sciences, Uniformed Services University of the Health Sciences, 4301 Jones Bridge Road, Bethesda, MD 20814, USA; [c] Department of Radiology, National Capital Consortium, Walter Reed National Military Medical Center, 8901 Rockville Pike, Building 9, 1st Floor, Bethesda, MD 20889, USA
* Corresponding author. Department of Radiology, Walter Reed NMMC, 8901 Rockville Pike, Building 9, 1st floor, Bethesda, MD 20889.
E-mail address: Paul.G.Peterson3.mil@mail.mil

INTRODUCTION

The American Heart Association[1] estimates that 92.1 million US adults have some form of cardiovascular disease (CVD). By 2030, CVD will affect nearly half of the US population. Public awareness and secondary prevention programs targeting behaviors (eg, exercise, smoking cessation programs, diet quality, and body mass index) and risk factors (eg, blood cholesterol, blood pressure, blood glucose) have modestly (6.7% reduction) impacted CVD-related deaths. Despite this, CVD remains the most common underlying cause of death and accounts for nearly one-third of global deaths. Many patients are asymptomatic until the late stages of disease when they present with acute, life-threatening disease. Early detection, risk assessment, and behavior/health-factor intervention are essential to lower CVD morbidity and mortality.

Computed tomography (CT) and MRI can provide valuable insight for risk assessment and management of patients with known or suspected CVD. Novel acquisition schemes and technological improvements have made coronary artery calcium (CAC) scoring CT, coronary CT angiography (CCTA), and cardiac MRI (CMR) more available and clinically practical for primary care practice. Reductions in CT radiation dose, rapid imaging techniques in CMR, and increased awareness have promoted CT and MRI use for detection and surveillance of CVD. Hardware and software developments allow for faster postprocessing and manipulation of large data sets, helping to answer key clinical questions with greater efficiency and accuracy. Manufacturing efficiencies have helped make CT and MRI technology more accessible at community hospitals. CT and CMR now rival echocardiography and nuclear medicine myocardial perfusion scans (nuclear stress tests) as mainstays of cardiac imaging for risk stratification and disease diagnosis. This article reviews current appropriateness criteria for CT and CMR, highlighting use in common clinical scenarios. Patient selection and safety concerns related to application of CT and CMR in the cardiovascular patient are also reviewed.

CARDIAC COMPUTED TOMOGRAPHY: CORONARY ARTERY CALCIUM SCORING AND CORONARY COMPUTED TOMOGRAPHY ANGIOGRAPHY

CAC has been a longstanding marker for the presence of coronary atherosclerotic disease (CAD).[2] Early attempts to identify CAC using traditional radiographs and x-ray fluoroscopy for early detection failed to gain traction, but the advent of modern cardiac CT with improved gating algorithms, faster acquisition schemes, and novel ionization radiation dose reduction strategies has made CT-based CAC scoring an available clinical option. Current technology enables CAC scoring with radiation doses of 0.37 to 1.0 mSv, an exposure that is similar to mammography (0.8 mSv).[3] CAC scoring can help target risk stratification and management of asymptomatic patients, particularly those at intermediate risk,[3] by serving as an adjunct to conventional risk assessment tools (eg, Framingham Risk Score). Although CAC helps assess the overall atherosclerotic plaque burden, it is not good for predicting coronary thrombosis (ie, "vulnerable plaque") or acute myocardial infarction.[2] Acute coronary artery thrombosis is typically associated with acute rupture of an atherosclerotic plaque with a thin fibrous cap or erosion of an atherosclerotic plaque. In both instances, atherosclerotic plaques are often "soft plaques" with little coronary calcium.

Modern technology and refinement in clinical imaging protocols have enabled the reliable use of high-quality CCTA in community hospitals. CCTA is rapid and has low patient radiation exposures. CCTA rivals conventional catheter angiography in the ability to illustrate the coronary artery anatomy. In selected patients, it offers a viable alternative to catheter angiography at lower cost and without the conventional risks associated with arterial catheter intervention. Unlike CT for CAC scoring, CCTA uses IV contrast agents to provide a luminogram of the coronary arteries. Contrast in the vessel allows for the identification of coronary artery narrowing and also helps outline "soft plaque" formation that is seen typically as arterial wall thickening. A recent meta-analysis suggests that CCTA is beneficial for CAD risk stratification.[4] Specifically, this review suggests that nonobstructive CAD detected on CCTA provides an opportunity to individualize patient management across gender and ethnicity.

CORONARY ARTERY CALCIUM SCORING
Technique

Calcium artery calcium scoring with CT uses cardiac gating to obtain motion-free, noncontrast images of the coronary arteries allowing for detection and quantification of CAC. The most commonly used (Agatston) scoring system, when combined with patient demographic data, allows for risk stratification that compares well with Multi-Ethnic Study of Atherosclerosis trial data[5,6] (**Figs. 1** and **2**).

Incidental Coronary Calcium on Noncardiac Chest Computed Tomography

Noncardiac gated, non-contrast-enhanced chest CT examinations can also detect coronary calcium. In these circumstances, conventional quantitative scoring methods do not apply. A recent practice guideline from the Society of Cardiovascular CT, however, supports reporting the presence of coronary calcium and outlines several qualitative and semiquantitative methods to do so.[7] It is important, therefore, to document the presence or absence and extent of CAC on CT scans of the chest performed for noncardiac indications. Used appropriately, these data may help with risk stratification.

Appropriate Use

The American College of Radiology (ACR) has appropriate use criteria for numerous clinical scenarios related to cardiovascular imaging. CAC CT is most frequently

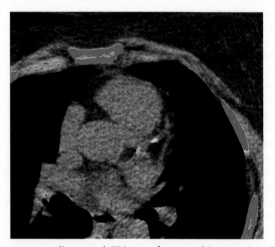

Fig. 1. Axial noncontrast cardiac gated CT image from a calcium scoring CT. Postprocessing software allows for color-coded coronary calcium scoring. In this image, the left main coronary artery (LM) is colored green and the left anterior descending (LAD) coronary artery is yellow. RCA, right coronary artery.

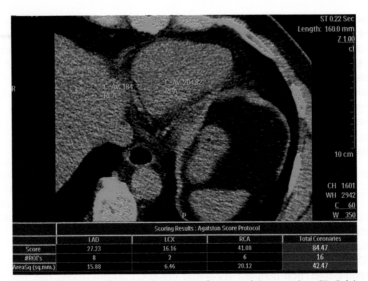

Fig. 2. Axial noncontrast cardiac-gated CT image from a calcium scoring CT. Calcium in the distal RCA is colored red with additional scoring data in chart below as is typically displayed for calcium scoring examinations. LAD, left anterior descending coronary artery; LCX, left circumflex coronary artery.

indicated in asymptomatic patients with intermediate risk of coronary artery disease (CAD). In some asymptomatic patients with low risk for CAD, a CAC CT may be appropriate in the setting of a strong family history.[8] CAC scoring is also helpful as a risk assessment tool for asymptomatic patients with diabetes.[9]

CORONARY COMPUTED TOMOGRAPHY ANGIOGRAPHY
Technique

CCTA is most helpful for coronary artery evaluation when both heart rate and rhythm are controlled. The typical goal is a heart rate of 50 to 60 beats per minute and normal sinus rhythm. Although protocols vary between institutions, oral metoprolol is typically administered 1-hour before the examination with the dose dependent on the patient's resting heart rate at the time of presentation (usually 50–100 mg). If the target heart rate is not achieved by the time of the examination, IV metoprolol can be administered if necessary. Unless contraindicated, sublingual nitroglycerin is also routinely administered immediately before the examination to aid in coronary artery dilation. Dilating the coronary arteries improves the sensitivity and specificity of the test for detecting coronary artery stenosis. Commonly, 400 to 800 μg (1–2 sprays) of sublingual nitroglycerin are administered within 5 minutes of the scan. Finally, a small test bolus of IV iodinated contrast agent is typically administered to determine the time-to-peak coronary artery enhancement, which varies according to heart rate, injection rate, injection volume, and access site. This "test run" helps verify the appropriate scan delay time after IV contrast injection and reduces nondiagnostic scans.

Imaging Challenges

CCTA requires a large-bore peripheral IV catheter (preferably 18–20 gauge in the right antecubital vein) capable of supporting high flow rates (4–7 mL/s). Standard examinations usually administer a total of 50 to 120 mL of IV contrast agent. Patients must be screened for contraindications to iodinated contrast agent, including history of severe contrast reaction or renal dysfunction before the examination.[10] Patients with a history of prior contrast agent reaction should be premedicated according to local institutional protocol or according to ACR recommendations.[10] In patients at increased risk for contrast-induced nephropathy, either an appropriate mitigation strategy (prehydration and avoidance of nephrotoxic medications before the examination) or alternative imaging modalities without IV contrast should be pursued. Relative contraindications to CCTA also include patient inability to follow breath-hold instructions and pregnancy.[11] Obesity and underlying arrhythmias are not absolute contraindications to CCTA, but may limit diagnostic accuracy.

Appropriate Use

CCTA is best used for symptomatic patients in the following clinical scenarios[12–17]:

- Acute nonspecific chest pain with a low probability of CAD
- Acute chest pain suggestive of acute coronary syndrome if the patient is low to intermediate risk for CAD with negative cardiac enzymes and electrocardiogram (ECG)
- Chronic chest pain with low to intermediate probability of CAD (particularly in patients with atypical chest pain suspected of having noncardiac causes)
- Chronic chest pain with high probability of CAD (invasive coronary angiography remains the gold standard in this patient population but CCTA can provide additional plaque analysis as well as morphologic and functional data)
- Dyspnea in heart failure patients if ischemia is not excluded (specificity of CCTA in high-risk patient populations is relatively low due to the frequency of other limiting factors, such as increased coronary calcium and coronary stents)
- Congenital heart disease (CCTA is a complement to echocardiography and can be particularly useful if coronary anomalies are suspected)

It is unclear whether CCTA is useful in asymptomatic patients with intermediate or low risk of CAD.[8]

Depending on the scan parameters, CCTA can also provide functional and perfusion data. In cases of congenital heart disease or nonischemic cardiomyopathy, cardiac CT with IV contrast can be used as an alternative or complementary examination for echocardiography or CMRI. This is particularly helpful in patients with certain implanted metallic devices that preclude MRI.

Radiation Dose

Radiation dose optimization is guided by the ALARA (As Low As Reasonably Achievable) principles. Typical effective radiation dose for CCTA ranges from less than 1 mSv to 10 mSv depending on technical and patient-related factors discussed later.[11] Numerous strategies are used to reduce radiation dose for CCTA. As one example, scan range is limited to the area of interest, usually the native coronary arteries rather than the entire chest. The fundamental CT parameters, tube potential (tube voltage, kV) and tube current (mA), are also tailored to each individual patient based on size. Weight-based and body mass index–adjusted protocols are available for each CT parameter. In addition, tube current can be modulated during the examination to reduce the dose delivered through thinner parts of the body. Finally, the use of prospective ECG triggering (tailored to the clinical presentation) helps maximize diagnostic information at the lowest possible dose of radiation. Prospective ECG triggering offers significant dose reduction (often <2 mSv), but also requires a lower heart rate and minimal beat-to-beat variability.[11] Retrospective ECG gating requires higher radiation dose and may be required in patients with high or irregular resting heart rates, or if functional data are required. In this case, ECG-based tube current modulation can reduce dose while still providing enough anatomic detail to quantify function.

Interpretation

CCTA interpretation begins with an overall evaluation of image quality to ensure adequate scan coverage and optimal contrast bolus timing. Images are reviewed in multiple planes on dedicated workstations with multiplanar (MPR) and curved MPR images along the entire course of each coronary artery. Each coronary artery segment is evaluated for noncalcified (**Fig. 3**), calcified, or mixed plaque (**Fig. 4**). The impact on luminal diameter is graded using a 0 to 5 scale (0, Normal: absence of plaque and no luminal stenosis; 1, Minimal: plaque with <25% stenosis; 2, Mild: 25% to 49% stenosis; 3, Moderate: 50% to 69% stenosis; 4, Severe: 70% to 99% stenosis; 5, Completely occluded).[18]

Obstructive CAD by CCTA is reported when there is 70% or greater stenosis in any coronary artery (**Fig. 5**) or 50% or greater stenosis in the left main coronary artery.

CARDIAC MRI: ONE-STOP SHOP?

Over the past 2 decades, a variety of innovations, including gradient technology, coil design, pulse sequence design, and automation of postprocessing software, have greatly advanced the utility of CMR. These improvements have sped up image acquisition and minimized the motion artifact associated with cardiorespiratory activity, making imaging of the heart a practical reality in clinical practice.[19] Compared with CT, MRI has the advantages of no ionizing radiation or iodinated contrast agents. It is important, however, to conduct a thorough patient screening to ensure MR safety. CMR is well suited for the assessment of CVD. Performed properly, MRI can provide excellent tissue characterization, functional assessment of ventricular wall motion,

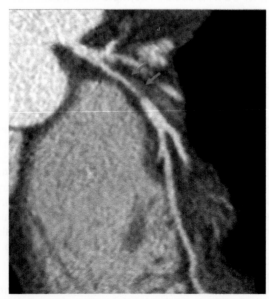

Fig. 3. Curved MPR cardiac-gated CCTA image revealing noncalcified plaque (*arrows*) in the proximal left anterior descending coronary artery.

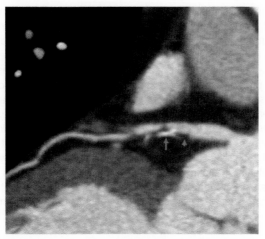

Fig. 4. Curved MPR cardiac-gated CCTA image in a 72-year-old man with atypical chest pain revealing a partially calcified plaque in the proximal LAD. Hyperdense calcified plaque (*arrow*) is located within a larger noncalcified plaque (*arrowhead*).

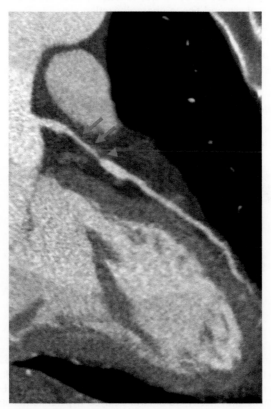

Fig. 5. Curved MPR cardiac-gated CCTA image in a 35-year-old man with left chest ache reveals noncalcified plaque in the proximal LAD (*arrows*) with focal 90% stenosis (*arrowhead*).

quantification of vascular flow, and delineation of vascular anatomy, potentially a "one-stop shop" for assessment of CVD. Cine MR provides accurate depiction of wall motion dysfunction in cases of acute or chronic myocardial infarction. T2-weighted images identify regions of myocardial edema in acute myocardial infarction. Using gadolinium-chelate contrast agents during pharmacologic stress and rest, first-pass myocardial perfusion CMR screens patients for potential myocardial ischemia. Dobutamine-stress CMR can identify at-risk ischemic regions as wall motion abnormalities in a manner similar to dobutamine-stress echocardiography. CMR also has the ability to identify myocardial viability as regions of myocardial infarction or scar that appear hyperenhanced on myocardial delayed enhancement (MDE) imaging (also known as late gadolinium enhancement imaging). Patients with greater than 50% left ventricular wall thickness hyperenhancement on MDE are unlikely to have clinically significant improvement following coronary revascularization procedures. CMR also helps to distinguish nonischemic causes for CVD that mimic symptomatic CAD.

CARDIAC MRI
Technique

CMR uses powerful magnetic fields and radiofrequency pulses to create images of the heart without the use of ionizing radiation. CMR is extremely flexible and provides excellent evaluation of cardiac structure, function (Video 1), and viability (**Fig. 6**) in addition to flow analysis and tissue characterization with T1, T2, and T2* mapping. As with all cardiac imaging technology, CMR continues to advance at a rapid pace, and defining appropriate utilization is evolving. The use of CMR for ischemic heart disease (ie, CAD) in an outpatient setting in symptomatic and asymptomatic patients and several nonischemic entities frequently encountered on CMR are discussed here in more detail.

Imaging Challenges and Patient Safety

CMR requires knowledge of advanced pulse sequences, complex anatomy, and pathology by both technologists and physicians alike.[20] CMR examinations take from

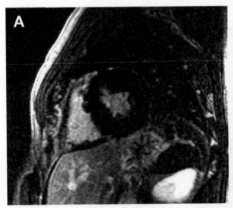 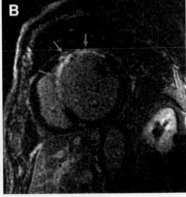

Fig. 6. (A) Normal left ventricular short-axis MDE image. Normal myocardial signal is nulled (*black*) to allow for better visualization of abnormal enhancement. (B) Abnormal late gadolinium enhancement with nearly transmural delayed hyperenhancement (bright signal instead of normal black myocardium) in the LV anterior wall and anteroseptum (*arrows*) consistent with left anterior descending territory infarct.

30 minutes to 2 hours to complete. The MRI scanner must be capable of obtaining fast, high-quality images to be of diagnostic use. A tunnel-type scanner with a field strength of 1.5 or 3.0 T is required to obtain images of sufficient quality to pass accreditation standards. The bulk of cardiac imaging has been on 1.5-T scanners, but with increased experience and optimization of protocols, the use of 3.0-T MR scanners for cardiac imaging is becoming more common.

As with all MRI scanners, patient anxiety (claustrophobia and anxiety regarding their possible diagnosis) can make imaging a challenge. It is generally preferred to perform CMR without sedation to the best image quality. Images are better if patients can cooperate with breath-holding and other instructions during the examination. Some patients, however, cannot tolerate CMR without sedation. Regardless of the medication used or level of sedation required, qualified personnel and monitoring must be on hand to immediately address any complications associated with the sedation procedure. Patients should be instructed to expect a long examination in advance.

Cardiac gating and breath-holding are the 2 ways to minimize motion artifacts on CMR. If a patient has a poor ECG tracing, irregular heart rhythm, breath-holding difficulty, or erratic breathing during the scan, imaging artifacts can be challenging to overcome. Although advanced techniques may be used to reduce respiratory artifacts, in general it is difficult to obtain quality images in sedated patients.

CMR patients must meet multiple MRI safety considerations before the examination. The Joint Commission recommends that practices follow the *American College of Radiology Guidance Document for Safe MR Practices: 2013* (https://www.acr.org/Quality-Safety/Radiology-Safety/MR-Safety). CMR uses ECG gating, can perform cardiac stress imaging in conjunction with pharmacologic stress agents, and involves the injection of contrast agents at high flow rates. Cardiac MR techniques require extra care and training to adequately obtain high-quality images. The use of advanced techniques and/or certain patients with medical devices require specialized personnel to be available to ensure safety.

Implanted Devices

An increasing number of cardiovascular implantable electronic devices (CIEDs) are being made to be used for patients with CVD. Cardiac pacemakers, implanted cardiac defibrillators, loop recorders, and other electronic devices pose several hazards. Lead migration, device/lead heating, arrhythmias, and the possibility of device malfunction are all possible with the use of CMR.[21,22] In some cases, fatalities have occurred from these devices.[23] Recently, MRI-conditional CIEDs have been developed. These MRI-conditional devices have strict guidelines for programming, scanning, monitoring, and interrogation to ensure patient safety. All implanted devices must be properly documented in the patient record for MRI staff to provide necessary safeguards.

Passive implanted devices such as metallic closures, stents, and filters are other potential safety concerns. In these cases, MRI conditions must match device-specific US Food & Drug Administration (FDA) approval parameters. Proper documentation of all devices (particularly soft tissue implants) is critical for patient safety in the context of MRI. Most orthopedic devices in bone, such as screws, plates, and many joint replacements, are routinely documented, but do not require manufacturer make and model. Large orthopedic devices (such as spinal rods) require additional manufacturer information to ensure patient safety.[24] Any passive device that has the ability to be adjusted via a magnet (eg, scoliosis rods, breast tissue expanders) must be queried by the MRI team before the examination.[24–26]

Even when safe to scan, implantable devices may cause image artifacts. Besides pacemakers and implantable cardioverter defibrillators, other devices such as pacer leads, prosthetic heart valves, and stents can also result in artifact that interferes with the ability to visualize key structures and accurately quantify chamber volumes. In addition to safety, scan optimization for artifact reduction is another reason information on all implanted devices is necessary before the CMR procedure.

Stress Testing

Cardiac pharmacologic stress using MRI has become increasingly more common. The most commonly used medications for CMR stress are regadenoson, adenosine, and dobutamine. Regadenoson and adenosine are vasodilators used for myocardial perfusion studies.[27–29] Dobutamine is a positive inotrope that is used for the wall motion studies.[30] Stress MRI requires the same level of patient safety monitoring as any other type of stress testing. Patients must be screened at least 24 hours before the study to allow for specific preprocedural instructions. Qualified personnel must be present in the MRI suite for stress testing. An advanced cardiac life support (ACLS)-certified physician must be present. ACLS-qualified nurses with MRI safety training should also be available to help with patient monitoring during the procedure. Following all stress procedures, a licensed provider must assess each patient before discharge.

MRI Contrast Agents

Nearly all MRI contrast agents are gadolinium based and predominantly cleared by the kidney. Gadolinium-based contrast agents (GBCAs) are well tolerated with few side effects. Patients with impaired renal function may be susceptible to nephrogenic systemic fibrosis (NSF), a rare, noncurable disease associated with GBCA use. The ACR recommends that individuals with estimated glomerular filtration rate (EGFR) less than 30 mL/min/1.73 m^2 not receive gadolinium-based contrast agents because they are at increased risk of NSF. The decision to use GBCAs in patients with low GFR should be done only if the potential benefit outweighs the risk and informed consent is obtained (https://www.acr.org/~/media/37D84428BF1D4E1B9A3A2918DA9E27A3.pdf).

Recently, patients receiving multiple doses of GBCAs have been found to have residual gadolinium in the brain. The mechanism of deposition, as well as any potential harm, is unclear. The FDA is investigating these gadolinium deposits, and a new black box warning in regards to the gadolinium retention (especially in children) has been recently released.[31] No link between gadolinium deposition and adverse health effects has been determined.

Appropriate Use

A large prospective trial comparing single-photon emission CT to stress perfusion CMR revealed that CMR had similar specificity and positive predictive value and better sensitivity for the diagnosis of clinically significant ischemic heart disease.[32] Both noninvasive imaging modalities reduce unnecessary invasive coronary angiography.[33]

In symptomatic patients with stable ischemic heart disease, stress CMR is appropriate in patients with high pretest probability of CAD. CMR is also appropriate in patients with intermediate pretest probability who are either unable to exercise or have an uninterpretable ECG.[16] Stress CMR is also appropriate in patients with newly diagnosed heart failure (systolic or diastolic) and arrhythmias such as sustained ventricular tachycardia (VT), ventricular fibrillation (VF), and exercise-induced VT or nonsustained VT in whom ischemic heart disease has not been excluded.[15] CMR without stress perfusion is appropriate for evaluating patients with dyspnea suspected to be of cardiac origin when ischemia is excluded and the examination can be tailored to evaluate for infiltrative, valvular, or pericardial disease. CMR may also be appropriate for patients with frequent premature ventricular contractions.[34] CMR is also useful in the

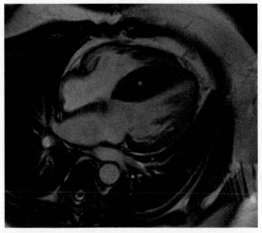

Fig. 7. Four-chamber steady-state free precession (bright blood) image at end-diastole in a patient with hypertrophic cardiomyopathy. Note the asymmetric septal wall thickening up to 35 mm (*asterisk*).

diagnosis and management of chronic heart failure to evaluate LV function in patients with technically limited echocardiograms.[35] In asymptomatic patients with a high pre-test probability of CAD, stress CMR may be appropriate if stress echocardiography is inconclusive.[8] Otherwise, stress CMR is not indicated in asymptomatic patients at low or intermediate risk of CAD.

Patients with nonischemic heart disease can present similarly to patients with ischemic heart disease. CMR is uniquely helpful in characterizing many of the nonischemic causes of heart disease. For example, if there is suspicion for myocarditis, CMR has become the examination of choice (when available) to evaluate for myocardial edema, early relative enhancement (hyperemia), and scar or fibrosis.[36,37] CMR is also the test of choice for evaluating infiltrative myocardial disease, including arrhythmogenic cardiomyopathy and hypertrophic cardiomyopathy, complementing echocardiography in evaluating adults with congenital heart disease[38] (**Fig. 7**).

SUMMARY

Cardiovascular imaging is an exciting and dynamic field with numerous clinical applications. Applied properly, cardiac CT and MRI can support CVD risk assessment, surveillance, and intervention. Well-established diagnostic modalities, such as echocardiogram and nuclear myocardial perfusion scans, are complemented by CAC scoring, CCTA, and CMR. In appropriately defined patients, these diagnostic modalities are useful for risk stratification, primary diagnosis, or surveillance. CCTA and CMR, in particular, are rapidly expanding in availability and accessibility. With increased clinical utilization and further improvements in imaging technology, the appropriate use of cardiac CT and MRI will continue to evolve, and knowledge of current appropriate-use criteria will help guide current clinical practice.

SUPPLEMENTARY DATA

Supplementary data related to this article can be found at https://doi.org/10.1016/j.pop.2017.10.006.

REFERENCES

1. Benjamin EJ, Blaha MJ, Chiuve SE, et al. American Heart Association Statistics Committee and Stroke Statistics Subcommittee. Heart disease and stroke statistics—2017 update: a report from the American Heart Association. Circulation 2017;135(10):e146–603.

2. Burke AP, Weber DK, Kolodgie FD, et al. Pathophysiology of calcium deposition in coronary arteries. Herz 2001;26(40):239–44.

3. Hecht HS. Coronary artery calcium scanning: past, present, and future. JACC Cardiovasc Imaging 2015;8(5):579–96.

4. Emami H, Takx RAP, Mayrhofer T, et al. Nonobstructive coronary artery disease by coronary CT angiography improves risk stratification and allocation of statin therapy. JACC Cardiovasc Imaging 2017;10(9):1031–8.

5. Agatston AS, Janowitz WR, Hildner FJ, et al. Quantification of coronary artery calcium using ultrafast computed tomography. J Am Coll Cardiol 1990;15(4): 827–32.

6. McClelland RL, Chung H, Detrano R, et al. Distribution of coronary artery calcium by race, gender, and age: results from the Multi-Ethnic Study of Atherosclerosis (MESA). Circulation 2006;113(1):30–7.

7. Hecht HS, Cronin P, Blaha MJ, et al. 2016 SCCT/STR guidelines for coronary artery calcium scoring of noncontrast noncardiac chest CT scans: a report of the Society of Cardiovascular Computed Tomography and Society of Thoracic Radiology. J Thorac Imaging 2017;32(5):W54–66.

8. Earls JP, Woodard PK, Abbara S, et al. ACR Appropriateness Criteria® Asymptompatic Patient at Risk for Coronary Artery Disease. American College of Radiology. Available at: https://acsearch.acr.org/docs/3082570/Narrative/. Accessed September 25, 2017.

9. Budoff MJ, Raggi P, Beller GA, et al. Noninvasive cardiovascular risk assessment of the asymptomatic diabetic patient: the imaging council of the American College of Cardiology. JACC Cardiovasc Imaging 2016;9(2):176–92.

10. Davenport MS, McDonald RJ, Asch D, et al. ACR Committee on Drugs and Contrast Media: ACR manual on contrast media. Version 10.3. Reston, VA: American College of Radiology; 2017. Available at: https://www.acr.org/Quality-Safety/Resources/Contrast-Manual. Accessed September 25, 2017.

11. Abbara S, Blanke P, Maroules CD, et al. SCCT guidelines for the performance and acquisition of coronary computed tomographic angiography: a report of the Society of Cardiovascular Computed Tomography Guidelines Committee: endorsed by the North American Society for Cardiovascular Imaging (NASCI). J Cardiovasc Comput Tomogr 2016;10(6):435–49.

12. Mammen L, Abbara S, Dorbala S, et al. ACR Appropriateness Criteria® Chest Pain Suggestive of Acute Coronary Syndrome. Available at: https://acsearch.acr.org/docs/69403/Narrative/. American College of Radiology. Accessed September 25, 2017.

13. Hoffmann U, Akers SR, Brown RK, et al. ACR Appropriateness Criteria® Acute Nonspecific Chest Pain-Low Probability of Coronary Artery Disease. Available at: https://acsearch.acr.org/docs/69401/Narrative/. American College of Radiology. Accessed September 25, 2017.

14. Woodard PK, White RD, Abbara S, et al. ACR Appropriateness Criteria® Chronic Chest Pain- Low to Intermediate Probability of Coronary Artery Disease. Available at: https://acsearch.acr.org/docs/69337/Narrative/. American College of Radiology. Accessed September 25, 2017.

15. Vogel-Claussen J, Elshafee ASM, Kirsch J, et al. ACR Appropriateness Criteria® Dyspnea-Suspected Cardiac Origin. Available at: https://acsearch.acr.org/docs/69407/Narrative/. American College of Radiology. Accessed September 25, 2017.
16. Akers SR, Panchal V, Ho VB, et al. ACR Appropriateness Criteria® Chronic Chest Pain-High Probability of Coronary Artery Disease. Available at: https://acsearch.acr.org/docs/69405/Narrative/. American College of Radiology. Accessed September 25, 2017.
17. Woodard P, Ho VB, Akers SR, et al. ACR Appropriateness Criteria® Known or Suspected Congenital Heart Disease in the Adult. Available at: https://acsearch.acr.org/docs/69355/Narrative/. American College of Radiology. Accessed September 25, 2017.
18. Leipsic J, Abbara S, Achenbach S, et al. SCCT guidelines for the interpretation and reporting of coronary CT angiography: a report of the Society of Cardiovascular Computed Tomography Guidelines Committee. J Cardiovasc Comput Tomogr 2014;8(5):342–58.
19. Ho VB, Reddy G, editors. Expert radiology series. Cardiovascular imaging. Philadelphia: Elsevier; 2011.
20. American College of Radiology, ACR–NASCI–SPR Practice Parameter for the Performance and Interpretation of Cardiac Magnetic Resonance Imaging (MRI). Available at: https://www.acr.org/~/media/61ECDDA970F34D58AD79A8657EAE1BFA.pdf. Accessed September 15, 2017.
21. Tandri H, Zviman MM, Wedan SR, et al. Determinants of gradient field-induced current in a pacemaker lead system in a magnetic resonance imaging environment. Heart Rhythm 2008;5(3):462–8.
22. Shinbane JS, Colletti PM, Shellock FG. MR in patients with pacemakers and ICDs: defining the issues. J Cardiovasc Magn Reson 2007;9(1):5–13.
23. Gimbel JR, Bailey SM, Tchou PJ, et al. Strategies for the safe magnetic resonance imaging of pacemaker-dependent patients. Pacing Clin Electrophysiol 2005;28(10):1041–6.
24. Shellock F. Reference manual for magnetic resonance safety, implants, and devices: 2017 edition. Los Angeles, CA: Biomedical Research Publishing Group; 2017.
25. Budd HR, Stokes OM, Meakin J, et al. Safety and compatibility of magnetic-controlled growing rods and magnetic resonance imaging. Eur Spine J 2016;25(2):578–82.
26. Thimmappa ND, Prince MR, Colen KL, et al. Breast tissue expanders with magnetic ports: clinical experience at 1.5 T. Plast Reconstr Surg 2016;138(6):1171–8.
27. Nguyen KL, Bandettini WP, Shanbhag S, et al. Safety and tolerability of regadenoson CMR. Eur Heart J Cardiovasc Imaging 2014;15(7):753–60.
28. Nagel E, Klein C, Paetsch I, et al. Magnetic resonance perfusion measurements for the noninvasive detection of coronary artery disease. Circulation 2003;108(4):432–7.
29. Gudmundsson P, Winter R, Dencker M, et al. Real-time perfusion adenosine stress echocardiography versus myocardial perfusion adenosine scintigraphy for the detection of myocardial ischaemia in patients with stable coronary artery disease. Clin Physiol Funct Imaging 2006;26(1):32–8.
30. Nagel E, Lehmkuhl HB, Bocksch W, et al. Noninvasive diagnosis of ischemia-induced wall motion abnormalities with the use of high-dose dobutamine stress MRI: comparison with dobutamine stress echocardiography. Circulation 1999;99(6):763–70.

31. U.S. Food and Drug Administration. Medical Imaging Drugs Advisory Committee Meeting Gadolinium Retention after Gadolinium Based Contrast Magnetic Resonance Imaging in Patients with Normal Renal Function, Briefing Document, September 8, 2017. Available at https://www.fda.gov/downloads/Advisory Committees/CommitteesMeetingMaterials/Drugs/MedicalImagingDrugsAdvisory Committee/UCM572848.pdf. Accessed December 5, 2017.

32. Greenwood JP, Maredia N, Younger JF, et al. Cardiovascular magnetic resonance and single-photon emission computed tomography for diagnosis of coronary heart disease (CE-MARC): a prospective trial. Lancet 2012;379(9814):453–60.

33. Greenwood JP, Ripley DP, Berry C, et al. Effect of care guided by cardiovascular magnetic resonance, myocardial perfusion scintigraphy, or NICE guidelines on subsequent unnecessary angiography rates: the CE-MARC 2 randomized clinical trial. JAMA 2016;316(10):1051–60.

34. Multimodality Writing Group for Stable Ischemic Heart Disease, Wolk MJ, Bailey SR, Doherty JU, et al. ACCF/AHA/ASE/ASNC/HFSA/HRS/SCAI/SCCT/ SCMR/STS 2013 multimodality appropriate use criteria for the detection and risk assessment of stable ischemic heart disease. J Card Fail 2014;20(2):65–90.

35. American College of Cardiology Foundation Task Force on Expert Consensus Documents, Hundley WG, Bluemke DA, Finn JP, et al. ACCF/ACR/AHA/NASCI/ SCMR 2010 expert consensus document on cardiovascular magnetic resonance: a report of the American College of Cardiology Foundation Task Force on Expert Consensus Documents. J Am Coll Cardiol 2010;55(23):2614–62.

36. Friedrich MG, Marcotte F. Cardiac magnetic resonance assessment of myocarditis. Circ Cardiovasc Imaging 2013;6(5):833–9.

37. Friedrich MG, Sechtem U, Schulz-Menger J, et al. Cardiovascular magnetic resonance in myocarditis: a JACC white paper. J Am Coll Cardiol 2009;53(17): 1475–87.

38. Mammen L, Woodard PK, Abbara S, et al. ACR Appropriateness Criteria® Non-ischemic Myocardial Disease with Clinical Manifestations (Ischemic Cardiomyopathy Already Excluded). American College of Radiology. Available at: https:// acsearch.acr.org/docs/3082580/Narrative/. Accessed September 25, 2017.

Printed and bound by CPI Group (UK) Ltd, Croydon, CR0 4YY

07/10/2024

01040500-0014